# PICTURE PERFECT WEIGHT LOSS

## *Shopper's Guide*

### Supermarket Choices
### for Permanent Weight Loss

## Dr. Howard M. Shapiro

RODALE

**Notice**
This book is intended as a reference volume only, not as a medical manual. The information given here is designed to help you make informed decisions about your health. It is not intended as a substitute for any treatment that may have been prescribed by your doctor. If you suspect that you have a medical problem, we urge you to seek competent medical help.

© 2001 by Dr. Howard M. Shapiro
Photographs © 2001 by Rodale Inc.

Printed in the United States of America
Rodale Inc. makes every effort to use acid-free ($\infty$), recycled paper (♻) .

Cover and interior design by Christina Gaugler
Cover and interior photographs by Kurt Wilson/Rodale Images

**Library of Congress Cataloging-in-Publication Data**

Shapiro, Howard M., date.
    Dr. Shapiro's picture perfect weight loss shopper's guide:
supermarket choices for permanent weight loss / Howard M. Shapiro.
        p.      cm.
    title: Picture perfect weight loss shopper's guide.
    title: Weight loss shopper's guide.
    Includes index.
    ISBN 1–57954–416–9 paperback
    1. Reducing diets.   2. Food habits.   I. Title: Picture perfect weight
loss shopper's guide.   II. Title: Weight loss shopper's guide.   III. Title.
    [DNLM: 1. Obesity—therapy—Popular Works.   2. Diet,
Reducing—Popular Works.   3. Food Analysis—Popular Works.
WD 212 S529d   2001]   1.
RM222.2 .S469   2001
613.2'5—dc21                                                            2001000246

**Distributed to the book trade by St. Martin's Press**

2   4   6   8   10   9   7   5   3   1   paperback

Visit us on the Web at www.preventionbookshelf.com, or call us toll-free at (800) 848-4735.

**To my mother**, Eleanor DeWalt, who at "a certain age" had the courage and optimism to marry again, and who continues to live every day with enthusiasm and laughter.

**To the many people** who have provided help and support for the *Shopper's Guide*, I am grateful.

Fran DeVito, the first to believe that Picture-Perfect Weight Loss should be a book, referred me to Carlo DeVito of Running Press, the second person to believe it should be a book, who referred me to Rodale Press, who have now made it two books. Without Fran and Carlo, not a word of mine would be in print.

Nor would these books have been possible without staff nutritionist Phyllis Roxland, whose expertise and conscientiousness keep me on-message; Susanna Margolis, whose creativity helps me convey the message; and Mel Berger, my agent at the William Morris Agency, who makes it all happen. Thanks also to Peter Igoe, Rodale's contracts guru, for his help and patience.

I am grateful to Gary Krebs, who began the task of editing the *Shopper's Guide*, and to Roz Siegel, who seamlessly picked up the thread and finished the job, for their expertise and unwavering encouragement. Thanks also to the entire Rodale team: copy editor Kathryn LeSage, researcher Teresa Yeykal, book designer Christina Gaugler, layout designer Daniel MacBride, photo editor James Gallucci, and developmental editor Amy Kovalski for devising, creating, and producing a book that manages to be user-friendly and elegant all at once.

Let me also express my gratitude to three public relations experts who have helped me carry the Picture-Perfect Weight Loss message around the country: Cindy Ratzlaff and Mary Lengle of Rodale, and Vanessa Menkes of Dan Klores Associates, Inc.

Finally, my thanks to the great Food Emporium supermarket chain for graciously allowing us to clog the aisles of several stores here in New York to do research and take photographs, and for being always welcoming to my staff and patients on learning tours.

# CONTENTS

## Chapter 1

# PICTURE-PERFECT WEIGHT LOSS STARTS AT THE SUPERMARKET

The first step to achieving Picture-Perfect Weight Loss is to focus on the food you buy. After all, you are what you eat. And what you eat starts with the choices you make when you go to the market. This guide will help you make the lower-calorie choices that take off the weight and lead to a lifetime of healthy eating.

During the course of this book, I'll go shopping with you. As we walk up and down the aisles of beverages, dairy foods, canned soups, condiments, and so on, I'll provide some overall pointers on what to look for and what to avoid in each food category. I'll even recommend some brands that I know to be particularly well-suited to a lifetime of healthy eating without gaining weight.

Pretty soon, as you continue to concentrate on

making deliberate choices in your shopping, buying the lower-calorie choice will become automatic. The information in this book will guide you on your way to routinely shopping and eating with awareness.

And awareness, as readers of my book *Dr. Shapiro's Picture Perfect Weight Loss* will remember, is the key to losing weight and keeping it off. Forever.

## Food Awareness Training

The acronym FAT spells *fat*. But the concept that it stands for, *Food Awareness Training*, is your ticket to losing the weight you want to lose. It's not about adhering to a specific diet or eating regimen. You don't have to eat six small meals 2 hours apart . . . or eat one large meal in the middle of the day . . . or avoid any food with sugar or fat . . . or eat mostly protein with no carbohydrates . . . or eat mostly carbohydrates with almost no protein. You won't need to constantly count your calories . . . or stuff a scale in your briefcase so you can measure the number of grams in a portion . . . or consult a sheet of paper reminding you to eat certain foods at certain times of the day or admonishing you not to combine certain foods. There's one basic problem with all such diets, treatments, and sets of rules and regulations: They don't work.

How could they? How could any single code of instructions work for everyone who wants to lose weight? We all lead different lives, follow different schedules, possess different body types, have different tastes. There are busy corporate execs who eat on the run and grab what they can when they can, calling it a meal. There are stay-at-home moms or, increasingly, telecommuters working in pajamas who find that being at home all day is an invitation to eat whatever is in the pantry and refrigerator. There are people who eat like birds and others who eat like vultures, people who love a huge breakfast and others who can stomach only a cup of tea in the morning, people-about-town who see stage shows 3 nights a week and follow them with rich restaurant meals at 11:00 P.M., folks whose idea of dinner is a pizza and a couple of beers.

If we put all these people on the same fad diet, what would happen? Assuming that they all stuck to it religiously, they would indeed lose weight at first: Any strictly adhered-to change in eating patterns is bound to cause an alteration in weight. But as anyone who has ever tried a diet knows perfectly well, the weight loss doesn't last. At the end of the diet, the weight comes back on. It stays there until the next fad diet comes along. Then there's the euphoria of another weight-loss success and the disappointment of the gain that follows. It's called yo-yo dieting, and it is emotionally unhealthy.

Rigidly uniform diets ultimately don't work simply because people aren't rigidly uniform. What's more, any food plan based on specific foods, portions, or times to eat is doomed to failure for the simple reason that it is based on deprivation. It aims to suppress your natural appetite—and, as with most things that are unnaturally suppressed, this only makes your craving more acute. When you do begin to eat again, you tend to do so ravenously.

The weight-loss program I've developed for my patients isn't a command to a robot. It isn't a regimen that tries to extinguish your natural appetite. Instead, it accepts the fact that you are an individual who cannot cancel every business lunch or refuse to partake of the family Thanksgiving meal because you are trying to lose weight. The program assumes that you have a life to live and an appetite that is part of who you are. The Picture-Perfect Weight Loss program asks you to be aware of what you're eating, focus on the foods you buy to eat, and make choices based on that awareness.

That's what Food Awareness Training is all about, and it is based on five core principles. Here they are.

**First, any reason for eating is okay.** When you want to eat, do so. Don't deprive yourself of food; it will just make you feel hungrier. Some diet regimens urge you to eat only when hungry. What does that mean? Do you have the time to analyze the early-infancy incident triggering the hunger of a certain moment? It doesn't matter what it is. If you feel that you want to eat, you really do want to eat. What you'll learn in this shopper's guide is to buy the lower-calorie, healthier choices *that you like* so that when you *are* hungry, you'll eat for weight loss—and be just as satisfied.

**Second, there are no bad foods.** Say it aloud to yourself: "There are no bad foods." This also means that there is no such thing as cheating and, even more to the point, no reason for guilt. Sometimes—if you're shopping for a birthday party, for example—only the chocolate-fudge mocha ice cream will do. At other times, there may be lower-calorie alternatives that are just as satisfying. But no food is inherently bad.

**Third, there are no correct portions.** If you can't fill a craving with one low-calorie frozen fudge bar, have another. And another. Even another. Believe it or not, with this particular choice, you're still on track in your weight-loss plan because, as it happens, frozen fudge bars are pretty low in calories. So if it takes a whole box of frozen fudge bars to satisfy that elusive thing called hunger, *that* is your correct portion. Hunger, after all, varies from person to person. Further, it can vary from day to day, even hour to hour, within a single person—something I'm sure you've experienced yourself.

**Fourth, an eating plan needs to suit your tastes and lifestyle.** Do you entertain a lot? Are you on the road 3 days out of 7? Do you have an endless commute due to which you're up and about and grabbing breakfast on the run at 5:00 in the morning? Are you part of a family of four with four different schedules that dictate that the only time you can all come together is for a late supper? Certainly, you cannot completely control these aspects of your life: job, family, obligations. But you can control the food choices you make within the framework of your tastes and lifestyle. Shopping for food is the front line of food choices.

**Fifth, you are not on a diet.** Ever. Instead, with Food Awareness Training, you're participating in an ongoing process of learning to make satisfying food choices. You make those choices at every meal, in every eating situation, and—first and foremost—when you shop for food. If you fill up your refrigerator and pantry with wisely chosen foods, you're already on the road to weight loss.

## What You Buy Is What You Eat

Awareness, to be sure, begins with seeing. That's why I call the program *Picture*-Perfect Weight Loss. It's all about the picture in front of your eyes, the food choices you see in front of you. The first place where you get that picture is the supermarket. Or it can be the deli, specialty shop, chain store, catering truck, or vending machine—anyplace where you buy food for your refrigerator, your pantry, your desk at work, or a weekend car trip on the road.

Whatever the purpose of your food shopping expedition, you will be confronted by numerous choices. In some of the megastores of today's world, in fact, the number of choices can be overwhelming. That variety is both bad news and good news for the weight-conscious: bad news because the variety can be confusing; good news because there are so many choices available that there are bound to be numerous lower-calorie choices. And it is the lower-calorie choices that are the key to weight loss.

Of course, the purveyors of fad diets would have us believe otherwise. They tout plans such as the high-protein diet, the low-protein diet, the drinking-person's diet, and the sugar-lover's diet. All these highly specialized approaches to losing weight simply obscure what every doctor and commonsensible layperson knows: that the only safe, effective, foolproof way to lose weight and keep it off for the long term is to eat a healthy, reduced-calorie diet and to exercise regularly.

Eat when you want, and eat as much as you want. But always try to eat the lower-calorie choice among food options. That is the Picture-Perfect Weight Loss program in a nutshell.

## A Matter of Choice

You're about to find out that you can eat a lot more than you're now eating and still take in fewer calories. You're about to see with your own eyes that it's okay to eat, even when you're trying to lose weight.

The **"Picture This"** food comparisons that you'll see scattered throughout this shopper's guide make it clear. They will help you see the impact of making the lower-calorie choice when you shop and when you eat. They won't just show you the caloric equivalents of foods; they'll also inform you about the nutritional values of the choices.

For example, perhaps you've tried to lose weight by giving up foods with fat, yet for some reason, the move to fat-free foods seemed to have no effect on what showed up on the scale. Why not? Being fat-free, whether inherently or because the food contains a fat substitute, says nothing about the food's calorie content. Angel food cake, for example, is inherently fat-free, yet it's high in refined carbohydrates that can easily turn to body fat if the calories aren't burned by energetic activity.

On the other hand, a plate of 15 assorted olives that are lush in appearance and rich in taste contains only 60 calories. And its fat content—yes, olives *do* have fat—consists of the very good kind of fat, the monounsaturated fats that we need for heart health. So, at fewer calories than a fat-free pretzel and with far higher nutritional content, the olives make a much better choice. The lesson? When you're in the market for a snack food or appetizer, think olives, not pretzels.

The suggestions and recommendations I'll offer when we go shopping in chapter 4 will do the same thing as the "Picture This" comparisons: show you the choices that are lower in calories and higher in nutritional value—the better choices when you're buying food.

## You're in Charge

In the end, it's all about your relationship with food. Awareness is the first step toward changing the relationship, and shopping for the food you eat is the first step toward lower-calorie, higher-nutrition choices.

It's in your hands. You're the one pushing the cart up and down the supermarket aisles. You're the one with the cash or credit card in your wallet. And you're the one with your very personal, specific eating habits and appetite.

Maybe you'll decide that when you shop you will avoid the high-calorie treats that you love, saving them instead for the occasional night out at a restaurant. Or perhaps you'll decide that it makes sense to

## Focus On
### Supermarket Saga

There are well over 30,000 supermarkets in the United States, most of them chain stores. The typical supermarket is nearly 40,000 square feet in size and stocks some 30 000 items. If you're a typical supermarket shopper, you're probably a female head of household, you make 2.2 trips to the market each week, and you spend nearly 9 percent of your weekly income on food (not all of it necessarily at the supermarket—less than the typical consumer in Canada or Japan.

buy a small amount of that high-calorie treat food to treat yourself occasionally.

Either way, you're not cheating on anybody. You're choosing for yourself. And the choices you take to the checkout register can lead to permanent Picture-Perfect Weight Loss.

## Chapter 2

# YOUR PICTURE-PERFECT PANTRY

*T*o change your relationship with food, you also have to change your relationship with food shopping. Since eating low calorie starts with shopping low calorie, each trip to the supermarket becomes an opportunity for you to assert that you're in charge of your relationship with food. Every time you toss a low-calorie food into the cart, you're taking responsibility for losing weight—even before you ever sit down to a meal.

There's a very simple formula for shopping low calorie. First, stock up on low-calorie staples for your pantry, freezer, and refrigerator—the basic packaged, canned, and frozen ingredients that you'll reach for to create tasty, healthful, low-calorie meals any season of the year, for any occasion. With these basics on hand, your shopping can focus on the fresh, *in-season* foods that complete a meal.

Let's put the formula into action.

## The Picture-Perfect Anytime List

The *Picture-Perfect Anytime List* is a menu of the lowest-calorie produce, soups, sauces, condiments, marinades, dressings, dips, candies, beverages, and desserts available. Stuff your pantry, refrigerator, and freezer with them and reach for them *anytime*. Feel free to go to the foods on the Anytime List when you want a snack or are planning a meal. Eat any amount of them for any reason. When the Anytime List becomes the core of your eating—in other words, the main dish around which you build your meals—you'll have no trouble staying thin for life.

Here are a few points about the Anytime List. First, you'll notice that a lot of it is taken up by sauces, condiments, and marinades. They're absolutely essential to your weight-loss goals and to your lifelong eating plan. The reason is simple: These ingredients add taste, flavor, excitement, and sheer pizzazz to your cooking and eating. Sauces, mustards, spices, herbs, and marinades can all make the same-old, same-old taste new again. They can enliven a bland dish, turn an ordinary meal into a gourmet feast, and change a so-so cook into an innovative chef. Experiment with them. Try out some that you've been reluctant to taste in the past. Let your imagination soar a bit. Think of sauces, condiments, and marinades as useful tools in the fight for variety, an essential ingredient in its own right for weight loss. (More about that later on.)

Second, soup is an important part of the Anytime List. This is not just because it is, as the saying goes, "a meal unto itself," but also because soups, like canned vegetables, have numerous uses in a broad range of recipes. Bring 'em on, and use them often to mix it up.

And speaking of vegetables, canned or otherwise, they too are multi-use foods. Today, a salad isn't only lettuce, it's also beans, potatoes, onions, radishes, carrots, pickled beets, marinated artichoke hearts, olives—a feast of colors, textures, and tastes. And for a main course, how about vegetables marinated in a special sauce of your own devising—flavored with mustards and spices, perhaps—then grilled on the barbecue for a superb summer dish or prepared on the broiler in the winter?

What I'm getting at with all these tips is that your eating program from now on should be a banquet of delicious tastes, a cornucopia of wonderful recipes that satisfy your palate while they contribute to weight control and your nutritional health. Keep in mind that the name of the game for achieving Picture-Perfect Weight Loss is choice. When you shop according to the Anytime List, you give yourself plenty of options from which to choose.

As a doctor, I think of the Anytime List as a prescription for weight control. Take it every day.

## The Anytime List

We'll get into more detail about each of these food categories and note some important points and exceptions later on when we go shopping in chapter 4. In general, however, my prescription is to keep these foods on hand and reach for them when hunger strikes. Take as needed.

### *Fruits and Vegetables*

All fruits and vegetables—raw, cooked, fresh, frozen, canned—belong on the Picture-Perfect Anytime List. Avoid any packaged fruits that have added sugar. Otherwise, the more fruits and vegetables you eat, the better.

### *Soups*

You've heard of value for money. Soups give you very good value for the calories. They are filling; a bowl of soup can be an entire meal. They are satisfying. For many people, they are more satisfying than raw vegetables, while they bring you all the benefits of vegetables. They are inexpensive, convenient, easy, and fast to make. Soups don't make you feel like you're on a diet. And above all, in my view, soups are versatile. They can serve as a snack, as part of a meal, or as a cooking ingredient.

### Sauces, Condiments, and Marinades

Put the following items at the very top of your shopping list. They're invaluable for adding flavor, moisture, texture, and versatility to every food and every meal.

- Salad dressings: oil-free or low-calorie (light or lite)
- Mayonnaise: nonfat or light
- Sour cream or yogurt: nonfat, plain or with NutraSweet; or nondairy substitutes for sour cream and yogurt
- Mustards: Dijon, Pommery, and other kinds
- Tomato purée, tomato paste, and tomato sauce
- Clam juice, tomato juice, V8 juice, and lemon or lime juice
- Butter Buds or Molly McButter
- Nonstick sprays (such as Pam) in butter, olive oil, garlic, or lemon flavors
- Vinegars: balsamic, cider, wine, tarragon, and so on

- Horseradish: red and white
- Sauces: salsa, cocktail sauce, tamari, soy sauce, A.1., Worcestershire sauce, barbecue sauce, ketchup, duck sauce, chutney, relish, and more
- Onion: fresh, juice, flakes, or powder
- Garlic: fresh, juice, flakes, or powder
- Herbs: any, including basil, oregano, tarragon, thyme, rosemary, marjoram, dill, chives, sage, bay leaves, and so on
- Spices: any, including cinnamon, cloves, ginger, cumin, nutmeg, coriander, curry, paprika, allspice, and so on
- Extracts: vanilla, almond, peppermint, maple, coconut, chocolate, and so on
- Soups as seasoning (see chapter 4 for more details and a couple of exceptions)

### Dressings and Dips

I recommend fat-free or light dressings and dips. The light category—low fat, reduced fat, or low calorie—is midway between totally fat-free and regular and is often more pleasing to the palate than fat-free. Dressings can be used as all-purpose condiments, as dips, toppings, even cooking liquids. They already contain a mixture of ingredients, so just slather them on vegetables, seafood, and pretty much anything else. Or cook with them to make up for the lack of butter or oil. I recommend keeping on hand several variations of dressings and dips, including at least one creamy version. Try brushing a light creamy dressing on seafood, then broiling; the dressing adds moisture and flavor.

### Candy

Yup, candy. The real thing—*not* the "dietetic" variety—is best when your sweet tooth starts aching. "Dietetic" candies have almost as many calories as regular candies, often lack flavor, and are an incentive to eat more. Stick to the real thing.

• Chewing gum or gumballs: any
• Hard candy: any, including sour balls, candy canes, lollipops such as Tootsie Pops or Blow Pops, Jolly Ranchers, Werther's Original, and TasteTations

### Frozen Desserts

Any nonfat frozen yogurt, frozen nondairy substitute, or sorbet is a fine addition to the freezer. Try the lower-calorie choices, among them:

• Soft-serve: up to 25 calories per ounce, as in Skimpy Treat, TCBY or Colombo nonfat frozen yogurt, and Tofutti

- Hard-pack: up to 450 calories per pint, as in Sharon's Sorbet, Low-Fat Tofutti, all Italian ices, and Sweet Nothings
- Frozen bars like Creamsicles, Fudgsicles, and Popsicles: up to 45 calories per bar, as in Welch's Fruit Juice Bars, Weight Watchers Smart Ones Orange Vanilla Treats, Tofutti Chocolate Fudge Treats, and Weight Watchers Smart Ones Chocolate Mousse, Dolly Madison Slender Treat Chocolate Mousse, and Yoplait
- Individually packaged frozen bars: up to 110 calories each, as in FrozFruit, Häagen-Dazs bars, and Starbucks Frappuccino Blended Coffee Bars

### Beverages

Avoid beverages labeled "naturally sweetened" or "fruit-juice sweetened," but help yourself to any of the following low-calorie beverages.

- Coffees and teas
- Diet teas: Crystal Light, diet Snapple, Diet Natural Lemon Nestea, Diet Mistic, and so on
- Noncaloric flavored waters
- Diet sodas: orange, chocolate, cherry-chocolate, cream, root beer, cola
- Seltzer: plain or flavored (check the calorie count if the product is labeled "naturally sweetened"; it usu-

> ## Calorie Caveat
> ### Little Aid from "-Ade"
>
> Heads up when you see a juice drink with the words "beverage," "cocktail," "drink," or "-ade" in the name, like cranberry juice cocktail or orangeade, for example. It's not real fruit juice. But even if it were, it has no fiber, won't fill you up, and is no doubt packed with calories. Choose water or a low-calorie beverage like Crystal Light lemonade instead—or eat a piece of fruit.

ally means that the product has sugar in one form or another)

- Hot-cocoa mixes: 20 to 50 calories per serving in Swiss Miss Diet and Fat-Free and Nestlé Carnation Diet and Fat-Free (avoid cocoa mixes with 60 or more calories per serving)
- Milkshake mixes: 80 calories per serving in Weight Watchers or 70 per serving in Alba

## Just Can Your Objections to Packaged Foods

The bulk of the Anytime List, as you can clearly see, is canned, packaged, or frozen foods. Somehow, to some people, that doesn't sound healthy or nutritious. Actually, packaged foods are an important part of your weight-loss eating plan—and they can be very good for you.

For one thing, foods that are frozen or processed for packaging are usually caught at their peak of freshness. What's more, the amount of nutrients lost in food processing is so minimal as to be almost nonexistent. And this minute loss is more than offset by the benefits, including having the foods there all year long and having them conveniently handy for any spur-of-the-moment hunger.

A can of vegetable-and-bean soup, for example, is a complete, healthy meal filled with just about all the nutrients that the vegetables would give you if they were fresh. A package of frozen raspberries offers the same rich vitamin-and-mineral content you would get from the fresh fruit as well as the same taste. And you can enjoy both of these items any time of year. In effect, the soup gives you all the rich taste and nutrition of garden beans and tomatoes, for example, and the frozen raspberries give you all the rich taste and nutrition of quintessential summer fruit right in the dead of winter. I call that very healthy indeed.

## Variety Is the Spice of Life

By letting you enjoy nutrition-rich fruits and vegetables all year round, canning, packaging, and freezing are good not only for your health but also for your tastebuds. They bring you a variety of tastes—and variety is an important weapon in the fight to stay thin.

Why is variety so important to weight loss? Because boredom is the great enemy. It's what makes people go off those fad diets: all protein or all pineapple or all something. Boredom is the "punishment" that tempts dieters to reward themselves with something deliciously high calorie because they "deserve" it after all that forced feeding of bland, tasteless food.

Boredom is never a problem in Picture-Perfect Weight Loss. Continue to refer to my Anytime List, a basic pantry for low-calorie eating. It offers a panorama of satisfying tastes, a richly textured portrait of varied flavors for varied palates. Packaged foods enable you to shop for this variety all year round. Eat them with gusto!

## Chapter 3

# HOW TO READ FOOD LABELS

*D*o you believe everything you read? Where food labels are concerned, you can certainly believe half—the half that's contained in the Nutrition Facts label required on just about all foods. The other half, the advertising taglines and slogans plastered all over the food packaging, is a different story altogether.

Let's start with the nutrition label. Food labeling has been a fact of life since 1973, when the Food and Drug Administration of the U.S. government first required it for foods with added nutrients or for those making a nutrition claim. The Nutrition Labeling and Education Act of 1990 expanded the requirement, making labeling mandatory for virtually all foods regulated by the government and making the food manufacturers responsible for the validity of the nutritional claims. Over the years, the label design has also changed so that the labels are easier to read and understand. The Daily Values measures are part of that; they're aimed at offering a threshold for defining nutrient content. To understand this better, read on.

## Nutrition Stats

It may be a good idea to find a jar, can, or package of food so that we can actually read through the label together.

The first and most important numbers on the label are right at the top: the serving size and the number of servings in the package or can or jar (not to be confused with recommended portions or anything of that kind; portions should be sized to match your appetite). Why is it important to understand the serving size and the number of servings in order to understand the label? Suppose you have a can of tuna. The serving size is 2 ounces, drained. The can, according to the label, contains 2½ servings. So if you're planning a lunch of tuna salad that uses the entire can, you need to adjust everything else on the label. If a single serving has 70 calories and 15 grams of protein, for example, your lunch is going to add up to 175 calories (2½ servings × 70 calories) and 37.5 grams of protein (2½ servings × 15 grams). And that's before you mix in the mayonnaise!

# Nutrition Facts

Serving Size 2 oz drained

Servings Per Container 2.5

**Amount Per Serving**

**Calories** 70      Calories from Fat 10

|  | % Daily Value* |
|---|---|
| **Total Fat** 1g | **2**% |
| Saturated Fat 0g | **0**% |
| **Cholesterol** 25mg | **8**% |
| **Sodium** 250mg | **10**% |
| **Total Carbohydrate** 0g | **0**% |
| Fiber 0g | **0**% |
| Sugars 0g | |
| **Protein** 15g | **27**% |

| Vitamin A 0% | • | Vitamin C 0% |
|---|---|---|
| Calcium 0% | • | Iron 0% |

* Percent Daily Values (DV) are based on a 2,000 calorie diet.

Note the relatively small serving size on this sample Nutrition Facts label from a can of tuna. If you eat more than 2 ounces, you'll need to adjust the nutrition information accordingly.

Or consider the label on your jar of peanut butter. It says a serving size consists of 2 tablespoons. That's *level* tablespoons, not heaping tablespoons. The point is, how many tablespoons do you spread on bread if you're making a peanut butter sandwich? If you use only 1, halve everything else you read on the label; if you use 4, double everything.

In other words, serving size is the basis for all the other information on the label, so it's the first thing you need to look at.

## Focus On
### The Great Peanut Butter Myth

Peanut butter—regular, not reduced-fat—is a heart-healthy food with almost none of the dangerous trans fat that increases your LDL, or "bad," cholesterol levels. Surprised? A plant food, peanut butter is cholesterol-free, it's low in saturated fat, and, as part of a low-saturated-fat diet, it can help lower the level of triglycerides (neutral fats) in your system. A tiny amount of trans fat prevents oil separation and maintains freshness. Reduced-fat peanut butter has about the same calorie count as regular peanut butter, contains more carbohydrates, and can lull you into permitting yourself to indulge on portion size.

Next, check out calories per serving. Notice that they're expressed as a plain number—72 calories for a 2-ounce serving of tuna, 190 calories for 2 tablespoons of peanut butter. Calories from fat are also just a number: 15 for the tuna, 146 for the peanut butter.

Just about everything else on the label, however, is expressed as a percentage of the Daily Values, or DV, even when it is also measured in grams. DVs are government-determined measurements that can be used as a general guide to a healthy diet. They are not recommended intakes; after all, an individual's nutritional requirements may be influenced by many factors. Rather, the DVs are reference points intended to give you some perspective on your overall daily dietary needs.

Nutrition labels are required to show the *percentages* of Daily Values of several key ingredients in the food. For the percentages to make sense, however, you first must know what the Daily Values for these nutritional requirements are. On the next page, you'll find the basic DVs, based on a benchmark diet of 2,000 calories per day. This is the number commonly used as the standard.

## Daily Nutritional Values

| | |
|---:|:---|
| Total fat | less than 65 g |
| Saturated fat | less than 20 g |
| Cholesterol | less than 300 mg |
| Sodium | less than 2,400 mg |
| Total carbohydrate | 300 g |
| Dietary fiber | 25 g |
| Potassium | 3,500 mg |
| Protein | 50 g |

Source: FDA

In addition to these measurements, nutrition labels must also measure the percentages of the DVs of vitamin A, vitamin C, calcium, and iron. And while not required, many labels add information about other vitamins, minerals, fats, fibers, sugars, carbohydrates, and even about alcohol.

It's important to keep in mind that DVs are general guidelines only. They're not meant as specific recommendations, and they don't tell you everything you need to know about what you're eating. For example, even if you take in less than the recommended DV of total fat, 65 grams, if it's the bad type of fat—the kind that raises your cholesterol and endangers your heart health—you're not doing yourself any good at all, in terms of either weight loss or all-around health.

## Focus On
### Fat and Cholesterol:
### Good Guys versus Bad Guys

Bad fats increase cholesterol levels, especially LDL, or "bad," cholesterol levels. Good fats can lower LDL cholesterol levels and maintain or even raise HDL, or "good," cholesterol.

| Bad Fats | Good Fats |
| --- | --- |
| Saturated (found in animal products, except fish; also found in palm and coconut oils, for example, in cocoa butter) | Monounsaturated (found in plant foods, for example, avocados; and canola oil, peanut oils, and olive oil) |
| Trans (found in many commercially packaged and fried foods, for example, shortenings and many margarines) | Polyunsaturated (found in plant foods, fatty fish, vegetable oils like corn oil, and nut and seed oils, for example, safflower oil) |

Still, the nutrition label can tell you a lot. It can help raise your awareness level and make you a more mindful low-calorie shopper. Make use of it.

## The Fudge Is in the Lingo

While nutrition labels are government mandated and monitored, the same cannot be said for the so-called information contained on the front part of a food package—the part thought up by the folks on Madison Avenue.

Let me put it simply: There's an awful lot of hooey in the descriptions and slogans splashed across the packages, jars, bottles, and cans in which our food is sold. No rules apply, and that seems to be practically an invitation to merchandisers and advertisers to fudge the facts.

Sometimes the words shouted out at you from the package are downright misleading. CHOLESTEROL-FREE POTATO CHIPS! the brightly colored package proclaims. Guess what. *No* potato chips have cholesterol; cholesterol is not found in any food that comes from a vegetable.

But freedom from cholesterol doesn't make potato chips healthy. On the contrary, many brands of potato chips contain just about the worst kind of fat that any food can have: trans fat. It comes from adding hydrogen to unsaturated vegetable oils to increase their shelf life, and it increases LDL cholesterol (the "bad" kind). For an extra demerit, it may actually decrease the HDL, or "good," cholesterol that you do need. As for calories, potato chips clock in at some 150 calories per ounce—hardly a caloric first choice. Even fat-free or baked potato chips are no bargain; I classify them as food saboteurs. (Read more about them in chapter 5.)

Here's another example of how the words on a food package may be a deliberate attempt to fudge the issue. Take a look at some of the so-called all-fruit, spreadable-fruit, or sweetened-with-fruit-juice jams and jellies. The impression you get is that you're spreading fruit on your bread, that you're sweetening your food with fruit rather than with sugar. The fact is, however, that sugar is sugar, whether it comes from fruit or the sugar bowl. What's more, many of these jams and jellies really consist mostly of fruit juice concentrate. And calories? At up to 40 calories per tablespoon, many of these spreads are not much lower in calorie count than regular jams, while offering no particular nutritional benefit.

Sometimes, advertising is accurate but utterly meaningless. My favorite is the use of the word *natural*. It's worn like a badge of honor, and it's meant to convey a sense of healthful nutrition.

Well, cholesterol is natural. Saturated fats are natural. Tobacco is natural. And not one of those natural substances is either healthy *or* nutritional. Natural *per se*, therefore, isn't necessarily desirable, nutritionally speaking. Nor do "natural ingredients" necessarily make the best choice for weight loss. How can you tell? Check out the calorie count. Chances are that the "naturally sweetened" cookie or beverage has the same number of calories as a cookie or drink made with refined sugar. You may as well consume the sugar-sweetened version—or think about getting your calories another way.

Another label that cries out for reading the fine print is "reduced fat." It sounds good, but once again, check the calories. To compensate for the lower fat, these foods are often loaded with sugar and other carbohydrates.

We'll look more closely at this marketing mayhem when we go on our shopping tour. We'll check out claims about "multigrain" breads at the bakery counter and "sugar-free" candies in the candy aisle. In fact, now that you're armed with the principles of Food Awareness Training, a crash course in label reading, and a skeptical attitude toward the advertising on food packages, it's time to head out for the supermarket and start shopping.

# Chapter 4

# Let's Go Shopping

*J*ust about everyone who comes to my weight-loss clinic in New York City is taken on a food shopping tour. From the corporate chief executive officer who has never set foot in a supermarket, to the housewife who is convinced that she knows everything there is to know about food shopping, to the busy lawyers and executives who say they're too busy to shop, to some of the most famous celebrities from the worlds of journalism and entertainment—people who are accustomed to picking up a phone when they want to shop—all of these individuals accompany one of our on-staff nutritionists to a nearby supermarket for a spin around the aisles.

Every one of them comes back with the full realization that weight loss starts with shopping, that taking control of what you eat begins with taking control of what you buy to eat, and that today's supermarkets are filled with choices for the weight conscious. In the words of one corporate executive who had literally never been in a modern supermarket: "These places leave you no excuse. Once you've made up your mind to take responsibility for your weight, you can't *not* eat healthful, low-calorie foods."

You've made up your mind. That's why we're going shopping.

## Some Supermarket Savvy

First, a few tips on how supermarkets work. You probably know that the fresh, in-season food is usually placed around the rim of the supermarket.

A financial motive also influences supermarket layout and the way foods are displayed. Staples are scattered everywhere so that you have to walk past alluring displays of the newest food release before you reach the frozen lima beans and can of soup that you went there to buy. High-markup foods are displayed at the end of the aisles because it takes longer to make the turn, so people notice those displays more than products on the long shelves. On the shelves, the higher-markup foods are those stacked at eye level— at about your waist level if they're foods for kids—so that those are the products you see first.

We're going to rise above all those gimmicks, however. We're here to search the shelves for the low-

BEVERAGES

calorie choices that can fill our larders and our stomachs with a varied, healthy eating plan aimed at weight loss and weight control. Not every product that I recommend will be available in every supermarket. But if a suggested product is a national brand, you can ask your grocer to stock it.

## Beverages

Let's start our tour with beverages—all except the alcoholic kind, that is. "Why beverages?" you may ask. For one thing, beverages are very often the first aisle you get to once you're through the supermarket door. A more compelling reason is that beverages are an easy category for the weight conscious because we can put advice about beverage shopping in a single, neat sentence: Don't waste calories by drinking them.

What do I mean by that? All juices, regular sodas, and the ever-widening array of flavored drinks on the shelves may be full of calories. Yet by their nature, beverages are an *addition* to a meal, or they're something you grab during the day just because you're thirsty. Neither is a good reason to waste calories. In both cases, you're far better off drinking water or a diet soda or low-calorie drink and consuming your calories in food. Rule of thumb? Chew your calories rather than drink them.

Here's an example: Suppose you have a craving for the taste of orange. Fine. Wonderful. Eat an orange. It contains as few as 30 calories, depending on the size and variety, and is filled with vitamins, minerals, and, of course, fiber—a major disease fighter and contributor of bulk. That means it helps fill you up and take the edge off your appetite. A moderate-size glass of orange juice, on the other hand, while certainly good for you, requires the juice from about four oranges—which amounts to 120 calories versus 30—and it won't fill you up at all. The lesson? When you want the taste of orange, eat an orange or reach for a *diet* orange beverage.

And as you reach for beverages on the shelves, do watch the labels. Beverages are one of those categories where the advertising lingo can be as misleading as it is enticing. For example, you'll see shelves of Snapple "all-natural juice drinks." They come in many exotic-sounding flavors, they sound healthy, and the bottles are enticing to look at. But the calorie count is high. Stick to diet Snapple, which also comes in a range of flavors, everything from cranberry raspberry to peach tea to pink lemonade to orange carrot.

Some beverages are now advertising added protein. Nantucket Super Nectars Protein Smooth, for example, promises health benefits, is marketed as a juice, and in that lengthy title seems to guarantee something for everyone. But at 280 calories per serving, you're better off getting the health benefits of protein elsewhere. As for the taste of a juice or smoothie, eat a piece of fruit instead.

Coffee and chocolate drinks are another subcategory where you're probably better off drinking the real thing. The Starbucks Frappuccino concoction, for example, makes the claim of being low fat. With only 3 grams of fat per serving, that's a fair claim. But the 190 calories per serving take this drink out of the running for a weight-loss choice, especially since those 190 calories come mainly from sugar. Instead, get yourself a real iced coffee and sweeten it with a low-calorie sweetener.

One more beverage caveat: Watch out for waters. Products like Splash or Clearly Canadian certainly look like water or sparkling water. They claim to contain "all-natural fruit flavors," many of which—like grape or blackberry—sound both delicious and healthful. The bottles are beautifully designed, graceful, easy to reach for. You wonder to yourself: How can this be bad?

Check the calorie count, and then check the ingredients list. At anywhere from 130 to 250 calories per bottle, these "waters" are not a good choice for the calorie conscious. With the ingredient lists showing fructose and/or corn syrup at virtually the top of the pile, you take in lots of sugar with your high-priced beverage. Look instead for brands like Poland Spring and Veryfine Fruit$_2$0: fewer than 15 calories per serving, without high-fructose corn syrup. After all, you're here for the low-calorie choice. When you simply must drink a flavored water, 15 calories beats 250 every time.

And if you think that tonic water—clear, transparent, and just a mixer, after all—is a low-calorie drink, think again. It contains 80 calories per cup. So by all means, look for the diet version with 0 calories, brought to you by the major tonic manufacturers, Schweppes and Canada Dry.

Yet even with all these warnings and restrictions, your choice of flavors and consistencies in beverages is enormous, with new products pouring out of the beverage companies seemingly every day. The variety of diet sodas and diet drinks today is staggering. Anybody who remembers the era of soda fountains will be thrilled to find diet root beer from Stewart's—remember the old root beer stands?—and old-fashioned diet cream soda from A&W, Dr. Brown's, and Barq's. For someone with a really sweet tooth, there's Canfield's Diet Chocolate Fudge soda or Canfield's Diet Cherry Chocolate Fudge soda. If you prefer fruit flavors, there's an alphabet of them, from black cherry to strawberry pineapple, not to mention orange sodas from Sunkist, Minute Maid, and Slice.

There are even diet drinks without NutraSweet, for those individuals who want to avoid it or who have been advised to avoid it. People with a disorder known as phenylketonuria, or PKU, should be aware of products containing NutraSweet, Equal, or aspartame. There are also anecdotal reports of minor problems including headaches due to NutraSweet consumption, but the government has yet to find it unsafe. The label will let you know if this ingredient is present. Diet-Rite, containing acesulfame-K and sucralose, is the breakthrough manufacturer on the no-NutraSweet front, and others are sure to follow.

Let's put it all together this way: Drink water or any of the no-calorie sparkling waters and flavored waters—seltzers and club sodas included—on the shelves. Pick from the vast array of tastes and consistencies represented by diet sodas, diet flavored waters, and other diet drinks. For calories, though, stick to food.

Here is a list of beverage choices for the weight conscious.

**BEVERAGES**

## RECOMMENDED
### Beverages

❏ Diet (or low-calorie or light) flavored drinks: diet Snapple, Diet Mistic, Crystal Light, and more, it seems, every day

❏ Diet sodas: any and all

❏ Diet iced teas: Lipton, of course, Snapple, Diet Natural Lemon Nestea, and other suppliers as well

❏ Waters: any zero-calorie brand, including Poland Spring, Deer Park, Dannon Natural Spring Water, Crystal Geyser Sparkling Mineral Water, Evian Natural Spring Water, Volvic, Perrier, and San Pellegrino

❏ Diet flavored waters: Poland Spring and Veryfine Fruit$_2$O, Vintage

As a postscript, don't forget drink mixes. Sometimes, only a hot cocoa or a milkshake will do. Just look for the following low-calorie brews.

❏ Hot-cocoa mixes: 20 to 50 calories per serving, as in Swiss Miss Diet and Fat-Free and Nestlé Carnation Diet and Fat-Free (avoid cocoa mixes with 60 calories or more)

❏ Milkshake mixes: 80 calories per serving in Weight Watchers or 70 per serving in Alba

## Cereals

We come around the corner from beverages, paying no attention to the end–of–the–aisle display promising a "special" on bagel chips, and find ourselves in the cereals department. Wow. If you thought the array of beverage products was staggering, it almost pales by comparison to the shelves packed from top to bottom with cereal boxes. Of course, choice is great. The problem with cereals, however, is that their range of ingredients and the variety of claims on their packages make them difficult to evaluate.

As a general rule, for example, I recommend cereals that are whole grain and/or high fiber. But my general rule is only a starting point; it doesn't cover everything. For example, Kellogg's Special K is not 100 percent whole grain. Yet it's very healthful and nutritious, and it's low in calories. Grape-Nuts—the "natural wheat" cereal—is, by contrast, fairly high in fiber but loaded with calories. At 210 calories per ½ cup, it's one of the densest cereals around. It's certainly nutritious, but it's not a good weight-loss choice. After all, have you ever had a breakfast consisting of ½ cup of cereal?

Among hot cereals, Wheatena and oatmeal are

## Focus On
### Fiber Fallacy

Eating Grape-Nuts in the morning for all that good fiber? Compare ½ cup of Grape-Nuts, at 210 calories and 5 grams of fiber, to ½ cup of Kellogg's All-Bran with Extra Fiber, with 50 calories and 15 grams of fiber. The All-Bran gives you much more fiber and many fewer calories. More for less is a good formula for both health and weight loss.

the prime examples of whole grain choices. Cream of Wheat and farina are not whole grain, but their calorie counts are equivalent to the whole grain cereals. If you have a taste for one or the other on a cold winter's morning, by all means, dig in.

Some cereals add sugar but actually have fewer calories than those without sugar. For example, Cheerios adds a little brown sugar but has fewer calories than Grape-Nuts, which has no sugar but four times as many calories. Many granola-like cereals—whole grain, healthful, and "natural"—can contain from 400 to 600 calories per cup and are as easy to munch from the box as to pour into a bowl. Even a number of lower-calorie whole grain cereals—General Mills's Basic 4 and Oatmeal Crisp,

## Picture This

| 1⅓ cups low-fat granola 440 calories | = | 4 cups Multi-Grain Cheerios 440 calories |

and Post Selects Great Grains, for example—are good to the taste and good for you, but they too are easy to snack on from the box. In these cases, it's so easy to rationalize the snacking that the cereals can actually become a problem for the weight conscious. The bottom line is cereal confusion: As opposed to beverages, there's no one single criterion for making the low-calorie choice.

What constitutes low calorie in cereals? Here's where you really have to be very careful to check serving size, which can range from ½ cup to ¾ cup to 1 cup. When equivalents are fairly measured, it turns out that the calorie range in cereals can run from 50 calories to as many as 500 calories per cup. Obviously, for Picture-Perfect Weight Loss, you want to focus on the low end of that range. So be sure to read the nutrition labels carefully as you make your comparisons.

Here are a few more points about cereals before I

give you my brand recommendations. First, bran is an excellent souce of fiber and therefore a particularly good ingredient for people concerned with weight loss, so look for cereals that have bran in the title or that advertise "bran added."

But look carefully at the calorie counts of these cereals. General Mills's Raisin Nut Bran, for example, is filled with wonderful ingredients, including bran. But it is high in sugar and, at 210 calories per cup, is no calorie bargain.

Similarly, be very wary of those wonderful granola or muesli cereals that contain bran along with nuts, coconut, seeds, dried fruit, and the like. The pictures on their packages make you think of mornings in the Swiss Alps, even if you've never been there. They're costly. They also claim, rightly, that they are filled with good sources of nutrients. Indeed they are. And they are delicious cereals, but their calorie counts are off the charts.

Another problem with these and other sweet cereals is that they lend themselves to snacking. It's easy to rationalize filling up on these "healthy" snacks because they are indeed so good for us. That's treacherous ground, however, as you'll learn in more detail in chapter 5 when we talk about food saboteurs. Suffice it to say, the calories in these snacking cereals are a high price to pay for nutrition we can find elsewhere.

So, what *should* you look for when searching for the low-calorie cereal choice? The general rule still applies: A whole grain or high-fiber cereal is the benchmark. After you've satisfied that standard, look for the cereal that appeals to your taste and your own nutritional needs at the lowest possible calorie count.

The choices are almost endless. And with cereals, as with beverages, the manufacturers seem to be staying up nights creating new products one after another. I've noticed that so-called women's cereals are the latest in the specialization trend. For a long time, we've seen kids' cereals that are more like games or entertainment than like food—cereals like Froot Loops and Frankenberry. Now we're seeing cereals that claim to be geared toward women. My advice: Check the nutrition and ingredients labels to see what's really going on inside the box. You've heard of "old wine in new bottles"? A "women's cereal" could just be similar to other enriched or fortified cereals in a new box. That's fine—unless you're paying extra, in both calories and money, for the "women's" designation.

SPREADS

Here are my picks for the low-calorie choices in cereals. I think you'll find that a lot of them are familiar old friends. *Note:* The serving sizes below are those listed on the packages.

## RECOMMENDED Cereals

- ❏ Cheerios: 110 calories and 3 grams of fiber per cup
- ❏ Kellogg's All-Bran with Extra Fiber: 50 calories and 15 grams of fiber per ½ cup
- ❏ Original Shredded Wheat: 80 calories and 2.5 grams of fiber per biscuit
- ❏ Fiber One: 60 calories and 14 grams of fiber per ½ cup
- ❏ Wheaties: 110 calories and 2 grams of fiber per cup
- ❏ Kellogg's Special K: 115 calories and 1 gram of fiber per cup
- ❏ Kellogg's Product 19: 110 calories and 1 gram of fiber per cup
- ❏ Whole Grain Total: 110 calories and 3 grams of fiber per ¾ cup

## Spreads

Often, just across from the cereals, you'll find the spreads—perhaps because they also figure prominently in breakfasts. Peanut butters, jams, honeys: There are a lot of misconceptions about these items. Let's take them one by one.

First of all, peanut butter. This much-maligned spread is, in fact, a perfectly healthy, highly nutritious food. Whether national brands such as Skippy, Jif, and Smucker's or those made for your local farmers' market, all peanut butters are virtually free of trans fat, the heart-health buster that is one of the bad fats. The minute amount of trans fat in peanut butter has been certified as well below the cutoff established by the Food and Drug Administration for labeling a product as "zero grams trans fat."

But it isn't only what peanut butter does not have that makes it healthy; it's what it *does* have. It contains niacin, folic acid, phosphorous, vitamin E, phytosterols—all the plant weapons that fight heart disease. In fact, studies show that a diet including peanuts and peanut butter can lower the risk of cardiovascular disease by 21 percent—versus a low-fat diet that decreases the risk by only 12 percent.

So what about calories? Well, to be sure, peanut butter has a high calorie count: 190 calories in a 2-tablespoon serving. But that is almost even with the calorie count of, say, butter, which has 200 to 220 calories in 2 tablespoons, contains the bad fats that

SPREADS

peanut butter does not have, and lacks the good fats that peanut butter gives you. In other words, between the two, peanut butter is the better choice of spread.

When you choose peanut butter, buy the real thing. So-called reduced-fat or lite peanut butters are basically a joke. The fact is, they have the same number of calories as regular peanut butter. Sugar-free peanut butter is even sillier since the amount of sugar in regular peanut butter is minimal. What's just as bad about these "dietetic" variants is that they are an incentive to indulge yourself. If you're going to indulge, do it with real peanut butter, and take in health and nutrition along with your calories.

By the way, the word *natural* on a peanut butter label assures you that the product is made from peanuts only, with or without salt. While it contains the same number of calories as regular peanut butter, I think it has a better taste.

Several soy nut butters are now available. They are similar in calories to peanut butter and are a healthier choice than butter or cream cheese.

Since it's hard to think about peanut butter without thinking about jams and jellies, my recommendation is to go for the lower-sugar versions, those that offer 10 to 40 calories per tablespoon versus the 50 to 60 calories per tablespoon in the "regular" jams. Smucker's Low Sugar and Light Sugar-Free, Knott's Light, and Polaner All Fruit are all recommended.

Honey is another popular spread, of course, and to most people, it smacks of delicious health—a nutritious replacement for sugar. Alas, it's nothing of the kind. Honey is actually more concentrated in sugar than sugar itself. It offers no particular health benefits over sugar. And at 60 calories per tablespoon, versus 50 for sugar, it's best avoided as much as possible by the weight conscious.

A note about Nutella, which was all the rage for a while. It's only nominally a hazelnut spread. While the label claims that you're eating "a blend of fresh hazelnuts, skim milk, and a hint of cocoa," the ingredients list shows sugar, peanut oil, and partially hydrogenated peanut oil before hazelnuts are even mentioned. At 160 calories in 2 tablespoons, this is no particular bargain. Once again, if you must spread something, you're better off with plain peanut butter.

## RECOMMENDED
### Spreads

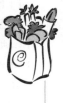

❏ Real peanut butter
❏ Low-sugar or sugar-free jams and jellies with 10
   to 40 calories per tablespoon

## Breads

Those spreads will need to be smeared on something, so we next head around the bend to the bread aisle, where the loaves are all lined up like soldiers.

Bread presents a fairly simple story for the weight conscious. Regular bread, whatever its type or flavor, clocks in at about 80 calories per ounce. If nutrition is your main aim, look for whole grain bread. It's rich in fiber—usually 2 to 3 grams per 1-ounce slice—and vitamins as well as taste. To find real whole grain bread, maintain a skeptical attitude toward the label lingo. "Multigrain," "traditional," "bountiful," and "natural" all sound swell, but the only way to be sure that a bread is whole grain is when the label says "100 percent whole."

If weight loss is your main aim, however, look for light breads. They boast only 40 to 45 calories per slice and come in a range of styles and flavors. While they're not whole grain, they do contain 1 to 3 grams of fiber per slice.

You will also see regular breads—not light—boasting 40 calories per slice. Almost always, however, these are exceptionally thin slices and therefore not comparable. Have a look, for example, at Pepperidge Farm Very Thin bread, with 40 calories in a razor-

## Picture This

| 2 bagels (2 sandwiches) 800 calories | = | ½ loaf of bread (10 slices) (5 sandwiches) 800 calories | = | 1 loaf light bread (20 slices) (10 sandwiches) 800 calories |
|---|---|---|---|---|

sharp sliver, against Pepperidge Farm Light Style, with 45 calories in a *real* slice of bread.

Just about all the major bread manufacturers make light breads, including Pepperidge Farm, Wonder, and Arnold. The last offers a particularly generous and varied range of flavors.

My recommendation? If you're having a sandwich, go for the low-calorie light breads. If you just need to sink your teeth into a piece of bread, consider the whole grain and take in the nutrition.

From these basic breads to biscuits, scones, cornbreads, muffins, and the like, it's uphill on the calorie scale. There are anywhere from 90 to 100 calories per ounce in all of them because of their fat content. At the top of the chart are croissants and brioches, with about 115 calories per ounce. They're the highest in fat—and it is the bad kind.

Bagels are in a class by themselves. Yes, in essence, they are low-fat bread, with 80 calories per ounce. The problem with bagels is their density. Because they're so fully packed and tightly wrapped, bagels are chock-full of calories.

Do you like a bit of bread for breakfast? Here's how some popular choices stack up.

| | |
|---|---|
| 2 slices light toast | 80 calories |
| 1 English muffin | 120 calories |
| 2 slices regular toast | 140 calories |
| 1 kaiser roll (2 oz) | 160 calories |
| 1 bagel (5 oz) | 400 calories |

Enough said?

## RECOMMENDED
### Breads

❑ Light breads with 40 to 45 calories per slice: oatmeal, premium white, wheat, rye, multigrain, sourdough, Italian
❑ Whole grain regular breads or rolls
❑ Pitas, English muffins, and other breads that may not be full-grain but are less than 200 calories

## Sauces, Condiments, and Marinades

Include in this catchall phrase everything from ketchup to glazes, from pickle relish to barbecue sauce, from plain old salt to exotic spices, from salsa to oyster sauce. Few categories of food are as important to your lifelong eating plan.

With sauces, condiments, and marinades, you indulge your appetite for taste, gratify your palate, and satisfy your stomach. There's a reason, after all, that variety is called the *spice* of life. The variety of spices, sauces, relishes, and seasonings on the shelves of your supermarket is what adds zest and flavor to your eating and your living.

I have a one-word recommendation for this category of food: Indulge! Calorie counting is not an issue here. The lower-fat sauces, condiments, and marinades can range from 2 to 40 calories per tablespoon if you do count. The point, however, is *not* to count. Instead, use as much as you need to make your food enjoyable to you. Even olives, which can run from 3 to 12 calories each, are rich in "good" fats. So I stick to my "Indulge!" recommendation.

Similarly, for those of you worried about salt, please be assured that it is a nonissue where weight loss is concerned. Of course, if there is a medical reason for you to restrict salt, you should certainly do so. You should also check with your physician before going in for salt substitutes, as they tend to be high in potassium.

SAUCES

So go for it. Explore the great variety of possibilities in flavor and taste sensation. In addition to the basic spices, the spice manufacturers make packaged seasoning mixes and blends. McCormick, for example, offers mixes with such enticing names as Key West, Santa Fe, and Monterey. Spice Island offers such packages as Louisiana Style Cajun Seasoning, while Knorr Aromat all-purpose seasoning combines numerous ingredients for you.

Experiment with the use of gherkins, olives, capers, pimientos, cherry peppers, and the like to turn up the temperature on salads or vegetable dishes.

Stretch your imagination beyond ketchup to include cocktail sauce, horseradish, Tabasco, Worcestershire sauce, hot sauce, salsa, and hot pepper relish.

Travel to the Far East—or to the Asian-specialties shelf in the condiments aisle—to find teriyaki sauce, hoisin sauce, tamari, oyster sauce, sweet-and-sour sauce, duck sauce, and black bean sauce for enlivening vegetable grills, seafood, or an array of salad possibilities.

If your idea of mustard is the standard yellow kind slathered on hot dogs in the ballpark, think again. Try Dijon mustard, Pommery, Creole, or the hot Colman's English mustard that you can either mix from powder or buy ready made. Your supermarket may also carry the original creations of local mustard makers. If not, prowl the next street fair, block party, or farmers' market in search of such concoctions as garlic mustard, horseradish mustard, champagne mustard, and the like.

Sauces and marinades: A lot of people assume that these should be avoided if weight loss is the primary goal. On the contrary, marinating adds flavor and moisture to foods—a big help if you're cooking low-fat. And dressing up your food with barbecue sauce, A.1. Steak Sauce, jerk marinade, fajita marinade, hickory sauce, chili sauce, or your own special blends adds taste for negligible calories. As for creating your own blends, try using any and all of the condiments and spices mentioned in this section, plus the dozens more on your supermarket shelves.

A note about cooking wines: They make fine seasonings (as do "real" wines) with no particular calorie impact because most of the calories are cooked off.

## RECOMMENDED
### Sauces

❏ Explore the variety of sauces, condiments, and marinades—and indulge

## Dips

You often find refrigerated dips next to or in the dairy section; other dips are scattered in various supermarket sections.

Among the refrigerated dips, many of the cream-based kinds are, in general, calorically deadly. What makes them that way is their high content of saturated or trans fat, which are also key culprits in raising bad cholesterol (LDL). Typical examples are Bison dips—for example, French onion—or Kraft's sweet and spicy barbecue, Heluva Good bacon and horseradish, Bachman's sour-cream-and-onion dip, and Wise or Frito-Lay cheese dips. Although these weigh in at 60 to 70 calories for a 2-tablespoon serving, which isn't so bad calorically speaking, most of the calories come from saturated or trans fats and are better avoided.

Refrigerated dips also include such favorites as hummus, made from chickpeas; guacamole, made from the nutrient-rich avocado; and baba ghannouj, made from eggplant. All are nutritious, with good ingredients and the right kind of fats, and all weigh in at approximately 50 to 60 calories per 2-tablespoon serving, which is only slightly higher than some low-fat salad dressings.

Among unrefrigerated dips, salsa is great nutritionally and calorically (only 10 calories per 2 tablespoons). Salsa also is available in a variety of flavors and heats. Look for Desert Pepper's array, ranging from Salsa Diablo to Salsa Divino. Or check out the choices from the Santa Barbara Olive Company, including roasted garlic. In addition, Coyote Cocina offers high-temperature green chili salsa and roasted corn and black bean salsa, among other varieties.

Bean dips are another good choice; they weigh in at 15 to 20 calories per tablespoon and have the added attraction of health benefits. (See "Beans" on page 73.) The same goes for light creamy salad dressings. You can read more about those in "Dressings and Oils" on page 69.

One more dip tip: avoid the cheese dips. They're heavy in both calories and bad fats.

## RECOMMENDED
### Dips

❏ Salsas, bean dips, light creamy salad dressings
❏ Hummus
❏ Tahini
❏ Baba ghannouj

## Rice and Pasta

In this category, let's include rice, rice mixes, pasta, couscous, polenta—all the starchy grain products. None of these come in a "diet" version; there's simply no such thing as "low-starch Carolina rice" or "lite linguini."

And there is no appreciable difference, calorie-wise, between packaged and fresh pasta nor between pasta and egg noodles. Yes, the egg noodles contain egg and thus some saturated fats and cholesterol, but the additions are minimal.

As for the vegetable pastas that are now so popular—spinach spaghetti, for example, or pumpkin linguini—the veggies make no difference in calorie count and, surprisingly, offer negligible nutritional advantage; they're there for the taste and color only.

Of course, taste is important, and the varieties offered in pastas and rices today are tremendous. Ronzoni alone offers tomato-basil linguini, roasted-garlic angel hair pasta, and garlic-and-herb fettuccine. DeCecco provides *tricolore* pasta in a range of pasta types, from skinny linguini to bow ties to tortellini; the tricolor of spinach, tomato, and regular wheat embraces the green, red, and white of the Italian flag. There are several dif-

RICE & PASTA

## Focus On
### Organic Foods

What is the exact meaning of the *organic* label on food products? According to recent legislation by the federal government, organic foods are not produced using irradiation or genetic engineering, and they cannot be grown in sewage sludge. Of course, we also expect organic foods to be free of synthetic fertilizers, pesticides, and chemical additives. (Nevertheless, be sure to wash thoroughly any produce that has not been cooked.) *Organic* doesn't necessarily mean more nutritious, either—especially if the organic product has been shipped from far away and has lost some freshness. One thing that the organic label *does* usually mean is "more expensive." So if you're willing to pay more for organic foods, be sure you're getting what you pay for.

ferent types of rice, such as basmati, arborio, jasmine, and black. Fantastic Foods as well as other well-known brands offers a wide range of ethnic accents.

But to gain real nutritional impact from rices and pastas, you need to search out the whole grain versions. While brown rice, which is whole grain, is a fairly common supermarket item, whole wheat pasta, whole wheat couscous, and whole grain polenta may be harder to find. There are some whole grain varieties out there, however. Look for Ancient Harvest quinoa pasta.

What are almost always whole grain are some of the more exotic ethnic entries in the rice/pasta field, the ones that come from different kinds of grain: kasha, or roasted buckwheat groats, an old Russian dish; quinoa, native to the Andes Mountains of South America; soba, a Japanese noodle made from buckwheat; and tabbouleh, made from bulgur wheat, a favorite Middle Eastern dish typically prepared with parsley, tomatoes, and spices. These used to be available only in health food stores, but their popularity is growing, and you can now find them easily in some larger supermarkets and in markets with large ethnic selections.

Given that rice and pasta are no carbohydrate-calorie bargains, what can we say about them for the weight conscious? Just this: To the extent you can, make these starches the third and smallest portion of your meal. Fill your plate and your stomach with vegetables, soup, and salad (seasoned to taste), then go for protein, and only then think in terms of starch. As we said at the beginning of this book, no food is bad, but if weight loss is your goal, there *are* priorities—and rice and pasta should not be at the top of your eating agenda.

RECOMMENDED
## Rice & Pasta

- ❏ Whole wheat/whole grain pastas: Hodgson Mill, Ancient Harvest
- ❏ Brown rice
- ❏ Other whole grains: quinoa, whole wheat couscous, whole grain cornmeal, kasha, bulgu⁻ wheat, barley, millet

## Soups

There are a million reasons why soups are a great recommendation for weight loss. Even though the calorie count can vary tremendously, from 5 to 300 calories per cup, so can the flavors and consistencies. That means the choices are almost endless, especially because you can mix and match different canned, dried, or prepared-mix soups to concoct your own creations. And whatever the creation, whatever the calorie count, the benefits of soup are tremendous. First of all, even a small cup of soup is a wonderful way to take in ingredients that you might not be so willing to eat otherwise—vegetables and beans, for example, with all their fiber and nutrients that are so important for your health as well as for your focus on weight loss.

In addition, of course, few foods are as convenient or as easy to prepare as soup. Even the most ham-handed amateur can open a can or package of soup. With some containers, you can actually pour hot water right into the package, and it's ready to eat. This means you can conveniently take soup to work for lunch or on the road for a healthful snack.

Soup's versatility is indeed one of its great virtues. As a snack, an appetizer, part of a meal, or the meal itself, the uses of soup are almost as varied as the choices of flavors and consistencies.

With all the choices available and with nutrition and convenience almost always assured, you barely need to check the calorie count when you shop for soup. Even many of the higher-calorie soups—most bean soups, for example—are so rich in nutritional benefits that, calorie for calorie, they're still good value.

There are two exceptions: first, soup in which the main ingredient is noodles or rice, rather than vegetables or beans; second, soup that is high in saturated or hydrogenated fat. In either case, you're better off making another choice. For example, you probably want to avoid lightweight packages of ramen—long, wavy rice vermicelli for soup that is originally from

China but particularly popular in Japan—and such convenience items as Nissin Cup Noodles.

You also want to avoid soups that get most of their calories from saturated fats like butter or cream; in other words, very creamy soups. Pepperidge Farm Vichysoisse, for example, is a thick-cream, very buttery soup. And while creaminess is not necessarily an indication of fat content—some soups are creamy due to puréed vegetables or beans—that is not the case with vichyssoise, cream of mushroom, seafood bisque, broccoli cheddar, or just about any cream soup. And precisely because there is such choice in soups, you can easily find other ways to stock your soup shelf. I've said that even the higher-calorie soup choices tend to be good values, but there is also an abundance of light and low-fat soups in an array of flavors, textures, and tastes. Health Valley fat-free soups, for example, range in flavor from corn-and-vegetable to lentil-and-carrot to a five-bean vegetable. Ranging from 70 to 160 calories per cup, these soups are wonderful weight-loss bargains. Even some of the chowders—Olde Cape Cod's corn chowder and oyster chowder, for example—come in low-fat or fat-free versions that are also low in calories yet high in taste.

And talk about convenience! Health Valley, Nile

SOUPS

Spice, and Fantastic all offer the pour-in-the-water containers with one-person servings of low-calorie flavors such as pasta Italiano and garden split pea (Health Valley), minestrone and lentil (Nile Spice), and chili olé and black bean (Fantastic).

There's even a whole new kind of waxed soup container that looks something like a 1-quart milk container; Imagine Foods has pioneered this packaging. As with milk, you need to pour out only the amount of Imagine soup that you want for each occasion, then you can store the rest until next time. What's more, the soups are highly nutritious. The organic creamy butternut squash variety weighs in at only 120 calories for 8 ounces, making it a major calorie value in the bargain.

As for soups promising "no added salt" or "low sodium," that is, once again, a total nonissue for weight loss. If you think there may be a health reason for you to cut down on sodium, check with your doctor; there is no reason as far as weight control is concerned.

The last ladleful on soup? Eat soup. It's good for you and good for getting to Picture-Perfect Weight Loss. Beware the fatty exceptions, but don't feel that you must restrict yourself to fat-free or light soups.

SOUPS

RECOMMENDED
### Soups

❑ All soups, whether packaged or canned, regular or
reduced fat/reduced calorie, with the exception of
noodle- or rice-based or cream soups, which are
high in saturated fats

## Frozen Meals

While supermarkets typically display all frozen foods
together, for our purposes it makes more sense to dis-
cuss foods by category. So as you stroll down the
frozen-food aisle and pass case after case of frozen
fruits and vegetables, remember that they are as good
as the fresh versions and belong on the Anytime List
of anyone seeking Picture-Perfect Weight Loss. Pass
by the frozen desserts and snacks too; we'll come to
them in due course. But do pause at the stacks and
stacks of frozen *meals*. This category includes frozen
breakfast foods and the frozen complete meals with
entrées and side dishes that are mostly sold as dinners
(although, of course, there's no reason why you can't
also eat them as lunches). Let's focus on them now.

And let's start with breakfast. Packages of frozen
waffles, pancakes, and French toast are a convenient,

quick way to get out of the house in the morning, and just about every familiar breakfast-food manufacturer offers these items. That includes Kellogg's, Aunt Jemima, Van's, and Pillsbury, to name some of the most familiar. Better yet, just about every familiar breakfast-food manufacturer offers a low-fat or low-calorie frozen version. Best of all, some of the versions offered—notably, those from Van's—are whole grain versions; these are both the healthiest and the lowest in calories. Van's whole grain toaster waffles, for example, weigh in at 155 calories for two waffles and are filled with all the nutrients that whole grains provide.

Eggo pancakes from Kellogg's, made without eggs, range from 150 calories for one blueberry pancake to 200 calories per chocolate chip pancake. Lacking the whole grain content, these are less sound nutritionally, but they are an acceptable calorie value in limited amounts.

If you love syrup on your pancakes, you're better off choosing the lite versions, such as those from Log Cabin and Aunt Jemima. They're usually found in the same general area as the regular syrups, but they contain half the number of calories. And they taste great.

Today's frozen-meal offerings are a far cry from the original TV dinners of long ago. In general, there is a great deal about them that deserves recommendation. They come in a wide range of meal content and include many ethnic varieties that present a range of tastes and textures. And the low-calorie kind, which I strongly endorse, provide good nutritional value conveniently and relatively cheaply.

My one reservation concerns the small vegetable-portion sizes. The solution? Add a vegetable side dish or salad, or precede your frozen meal with a cup or bowl of vegetable-rich soup.

Your best nutrition and calorie bets in frozen meals are those that focus on vegetables, beans, or seafood. The major low-calorie brands—Healthy Choice, Weight Watchers Smart Ones, and Lean Cuisine—are all fine choices. But be sure to check out the ever-widening range of ethnic frozen meals. Tai Gourmet, for example, offers a hearty, lightly spiced, tasty vegetable korma at 300 calories for the full meal. This meal provides a variety of vegetables and, of course, the curry taste of India's korma-style cooking, combining a touch of coconut, cardamom, ginger, cloves, cinnamon, bay leaves, and salt.

Don't neglect the ethnic meals being marketed by such homegrown food giants as Stouffer's Lean Cuisine, with Asian noodle stir fry at 240 calories for the package, Mexican tamale pie at 220 calories, tofu vegetable lasagna for 300 calories, cannelloni with vegetables at 350 calories, Santa Fe–style rice and beans at 300 calories, three-bean chili at 250, or vegetable eggroll at 300 calories. Or try Celentano's low-fat lasagna at 260 calories, low-fat manicotti at 250, and low-fat stuffed shells also at 250.

If I were asked to single out one brand, I would not hesitate to recommend Amy's. The variety is wide, the focus on vegetables is healthful, the calorie count is just right. Try Amy's Shepherd's Pie, for example, at a mere 160 calories. It's filled with nutrition, a good filler-upper, and very tasty indeed. It works as either a side dish or a complete meal—a good buy and a good selection.

## RECOMMENDED
### Frozen Meals

❏ Low-calorie frozen breakfast foods: those offered by Kellogg's, Aunt Jemima, and Pillsbury, with a special mention for the low-calorie, whole grain offerings from Van's

❏ Low-calorie, vegetable-focused frozen meals in the 150- to 350-calories-per-package range, especially Amy's

## Dressings and Oils

All the unsaturated oils are good foods, nutritionally speaking, whether monounsaturated, like olive oil, or polyunsaturated, like corn and safflower oils. (Saturated "oils" like coconut and palm are not true oils because they are not liquid at room temperature.) All oils also have 120 to 125 calories per tablespoon, the same count as any fat, solid or liquid. When you see a jar of olive oil labeled "light," that refers only to its color or flavor; light olive oil has no fewer calories than regular olive oil.

Oils contain the good kind of fat that is essential in a diet. The problem is that at about 120 calories per tablespoon, oils are also a very concentrated source of calories. For the person who is both health and weight conscious, therefore, oil poses a slippery dilemma: It provides essential fats in a good, useful, tasty form, but this benefit comes at a high cost in calories.

My recommendation? Don't bend over backward to either include oil in your diet or exclude it. Since oil is just one of the foods from which you can obtain the needed good fats, you can alternate among the various options: olive oil on salad one day, an avocado

DRESSINGS & OILS

# Focus On
## Seasoning Savvy

What's best for enhancing the taste of the food choices for Picture-Perfect Weight Loss? Try these tips.

| On . . . | Try . . . |
| --- | --- |
| Broccoli | Caraway seeds, oregano, tarragon |
| Brussels sprouts | Caraway seeds, celery seed, thyme |
| Carrots | Allspice, dill, ginger, nutmeg, oregano, parsley, thyme |
| Cauliflower | Caraway seeds, parsley, tarragon |
| Fish | Basil, dill, parsley, tarragon |
| Green beans | Basil, oregano, tarragon, thyme |
| Lentils | Cumin |
| Peas | Basil, dill, oregano, rosemary, tarragon, thyme |
| Potatoes | Caraway seeds, dill, fennel, parsley, tarragon, thyme |
| Spinach | Basil, nutmeg, oregano, rosemary, tarragon |
| Summer squash | Basil, fennel, oregano, parsley, tarragon |
| Sweet potatoes | Cinnamon, cloves, ginger, nutmeg |
| Tomatoes | Basil, cumin, oregano, tarragon, thyme |

Also try combining herbs and spices with sauces and condiments. For example, enhance a baked potato with light creamy ranch dressing topped with dill. Or make a tomato salad by adding basil to a balsamic vinaigrette. Experiment, be creative!

the next day, a handful of nuts the day after that, maybe a salmon dinner on the following day.

For those bent on weight loss, keep the calorie count in mind when you use oil on a salad or in cooking. You can get plenty of flavor out of a single tablespoon or even ½ tablespoon. And consider alternatives. Ready-made dressings or dressing mixes are a terrific choice for the weight conscious, not just as a substitute for high-calorie oils but also as a highly recommended food-preparation ingredient. They come in three categories: regular dressings, which weigh in at 60 to 90 calories per tablespoon; light or reduced-fat dressings, with approximately 15 to 50 calories per tablespoon, and fat-free dressings, at 2 to 15 calories per tablespoon.

Most of the brand name manufacturers offer all three categories in a range of flavors and flavor combinations. I'm hard pressed to find much difference in taste between the light lower-calorie versions and the real thing, probably because the lights have the same ingredients but lower proportions of fat. The taste difference between regular salad dressing and most fat-free versions is noticeable to many people, but these fat-free dressings are extremely useful as cooking ingredients and marinades.

DRESSINGS & OILS

DRESSINGS & OILS

## Picture This

| 1 jar regular mayonnaise | = | 2 jars light mayonnaise | = | 4 jars fat-free mayonnaise |
|---|---|---|---|---|

With the light dressings so numerous and varied, however, and with their calorie counts about half those of regular oils, it makes sense to get your salad dressing hit with such light ready mades as Kraft's Light Done Right! Italian, Light Thousand Island, or Light Raspberry Vinaigrette dressings. Or try Wish-Bone Just 2 Good! products, offering just 2 grams of fat per serving in such flavors as Country Italian with Herbs and even Creamy Caesar. A new entry in the field is Hellmann's Citrus Splash, light dressings in orange, tangerine, and other sweet-and-pungent flavors at only 90 calories for 2 tablespoons.

But the great bonus of the light or fat-free dressings is their use as a food-preparation ingredient. Take a lower-calorie ranch dressing, for example, and brush it on a potato you're about to roast or bake. Or daub light Italian on shrimp for the grill. Or use light creamy dressing right out of the bottle as a dip for crudités. The results are delicious and varied, and these tastes are gained at a highly affordable price in calories.

Here's another idea that's particularly well-suited to those trying to shed pounds: Think about using flavored vinegars alone as salad dressings or cooking ingredients. The taste range in vinegars is staggering—balsamic, pear, malt, melon, champagne, rosemary, roasted pepper, and garlic, to name just a few. At 2 to 10 calories per tablespoon, you really can't go wrong.

RECOMMENDED
**Dressings & Oils**

❏ Light ready-made dressings, on salads or in cooking: all national or local brands
❏ Flavored vinegars used as dressings
❏ All unsaturated oils, used sparingly

**BEANS**

## Beans

One of the three protein-food categories that I recommend, along with seafood and soy products, beans are among the most nutritious foods in existence. That goes for canned beans as well as the dried beans that should be soaked and washed before cooking. And, of course, canned beans win hands down when it comes to convenience.

But whether the beans you eat have been soaked

overnight or pulled down from the shelf on the spur of the moment, they're a particularly good choice for the weight-conscious. They're a good protein food that is rich in nutrients, filling, and, with a wide range of flavors and styles, appealing to just about every taste. That's why beans rate a special section in this chapter and have a whole shelf to themselves in the supermarket.

Just consider the options in the legume family: black beans, kidney beans, chickpeas, black-eyed peas, pigeon peas, cannellini beans, lentils, red lentils, split peas all line the shelves. And those are just basic beans. Keep on exploring the beans section in your supermarket, and you'll find an array of canned or packaged bean dishes, especially canned bean chilis. Check out Health Valley's spiced black bean chili or milder three-bean chili. Note that other manufacturers also offer a range of temperatures (hot, medium, and mild) in their chili-and-bean combinations.

Where refried beans are concerned, however, it's wise to exercise some caution. After all, as the name makes clear, this is a food that has been fried twice. That means twice as much lard for frying and twice as much fat—the bad kind of fat, at that. So go for the low-fat or fat-free versions of refried beans, with about 140 calories per ½ cup for the low fat and 110 calories per ½ cup for the fat-free.

That one caveat aside, however, make beans a part of your meal or its centerpiece, and you'll be on your way to Picture-Perfect Weight Loss.

## RECOMMENDED
### Beans

❑ All beans, dried or canned
❑ Health Valley canned bean-chili combinations
❑ Low-fat or fat-free refried beans

## Produce and Fresh Food

If you've ever been on a diet, you've probably been warned to distinguish between high-starch and low-starch vegetables and high-sugar and low-sugar fruits. Eat lettuce, not corn, you've no doubt been told; stay away from bananas and cherries, and stick to strawberries or melon. The reasoning? According to these other diet gurus and weight-loss programs, the higher-carbohydrate fruits and vegetables are also higher in calories.

Yes, they are. Slightly. But that slight difference in calories does not necessarily make the lower-carbohydrate fruits and vegetables better choices for weight loss. All fruits and vegetables are excellent sources of fiber and therefore good buys for the calories. Fiber is particularly important to weight loss because it fills you up and takes the edge off your appetite.

So forget about distinguishing between high-

## Focus On
### Winter Squash

If you're looking for a food that is low calorie, tasty, filling, and very, very good for you, stop searching: Winter squash fills the bill. It's ready when all the summer vegetables have faded and comes in many varieties: acorn, butternut, hubbard, delicata, buttercup, pumpkin, and kabocha (also known as chestnut squash or Japanese pumpkin).

What's more, you can bake it, grill it, boil and mash it, or—thanks to its creamy consistency—purée it or put it in soup.

Frozen winter squash is available all year round. A canned version is Libby's Pumpkin, solid-packed as a purée. Look for it among the baking ingredients, not on the vegetable shelf.

As for nutrition, a single cup of squash provides 10 grams of fiber, one-fifth of your daily requirement for iron, and more than 300 percent of the daily requirement for vitamin A, occurring here in the form of beta-carotene, an important antioxidant. All this at a cost of only 60 to 80 calories.

PRODUCE

## Focus On
### Taking Broccoli to Heart

Does broccoli help prevent heart disease? One study showed that women who ate the green vegetable at least weekly had half the heart disease risk of women who did not. Researchers aren't yet sure why, but the focus is on broccoli's flavonoids, one of the circulation-boosting, disease-fighting phytochemicals. Don't over-cook broccoli, though. Past the tender stage, some of its nutrients get lost.

starch peas and low-starch broccoli or between high-sugar grapes and low-sugar grapefruit. Instead, as you roam the outer edges of your supermarket, your eyes feasting on the rich variety of colors and textures of fresh fruits and produce, shop for what you love to eat. Everything you see is good for you. It's good for your health, and it's good for losing weight or maintaining the healthy weight you've achieved.

Everything before you—from the tiniest grape to the largest watermelon, from the fattest squash to the thinnest bean—is packed with the fiber, vitamins, minerals, and phytochemicals that fight disease and help you stay healthy for life. Variety and choice are your watchwords. By having such a wide and rich choice, by letting your palate as well as your eyes feast on all this variety, you will actually lower your calorie intake over time.

So indulge your taste for any and all fresh fruits and vegetables. Your mother was right: They *are* good for you. And they're especially good for achieving Picture-Perfect Weight Loss.

### RECOMMENDED
### Produce

All fresh fruits and vegetables, anytime, for any occasion, for any reason—without exception.

## Snacks

It's hard to live life without the occasional snack, and no one expects you to. But snacking—particularly on the starchy, crunchy snacks we all love—has a way of getting out of control. That small bowl of pretzels you keep dipping into as you're having a cocktail in the evening . . . the packaged crackers a coworker keeps on her desk, readily available to anyone passing by . . . the tub of popcorn that is an essential part of the ritual when you go to the movies. These munchies become such automatic reactions that we don't think about them even as we're eating them.

SNACKS

But Picture-Perfect Weight Loss is all about Food Awareness and the choices you make as a result of that awareness. Your choices are what will make the difference, whether it's at a five-course banquet in a lavish restaurant or at the vending machine in the office when you're looking for an afternoon energy boost.

The Picture-Perfect Anytime List back in chapter 2 offers lots of foods that make good snacks: fruits or candies or desserts when you yearn for something sweet, vegetables with dip or pickles or even soups

## Focus On
### Corn Calculus

As a vegetable, how does corn measure up?

First of all, it's not a vegetable but a grain, like wheat. Corn is chock-full of disease-fighting phytochemicals and may prove particularly useful in keeping your vision healthy. Corn oil also provides essential fatty acids and, in moderation, is a good choice for cooking and for salad dressings.

As for popcorn, it's a low-fat, low-calorie snack if it's air-popped. The movie-theater variety, however, tends to be packed with hydrogenated vegetable oil, a heart buster if ever there was one.

when you yearn for something salty. So when you're shopping for snacks in the supermarket, keep this in mind: Sweet or salty, an average serving of a starchy snack that is not on the Anytime List is going to be a lot costlier in terms of calories than a snack that *is* on the Anytime List. Put another way, if you choose snacks from the Anytime List, you can eat them until you feel satisfied; if you choose snacks not on the list, you're taking in a lot more calories—probably a few hundred more per average snack serving.

The problem with pretzels, crackers, and popcorn—all of which, by the way, are low-fat foods—is not so much their calorie counts, which are 110 to 120 calories per ounce, but the fact that it's very difficult to stop at 1 ounce. The average serving that will satisfy your taste for something crunchy will be a good deal more than 1 ounce. That means it will cost you a few hundred calories more than the possible snack foods on the Anytime List.

Of course, the truth is that even a bathtub full of vegetables won't do if what you hanker for is a bowl of popcorn. Sometimes, only popcorn will do. But there *are* lower-calorie alternatives to that yearning for a snack. Your supermarket carries those alternatives in the fresh-produce bin, on the dried-fruit shelf, in the pickle aisle, in the cans and packages of soups, even in the candy section. The choice, as always, is yours.

## RECOMMENDED Snacks

❏ Eat starchy, crunchy snacks only in conjunction with a food from the Anytime List: fruit with popcorn, soup with crackers, a few pickles with a pretzel; fill up on the former, and go easy on the starchy snack

## Candy

Candy in a shopper's guide to Picture-Perfect Weight Loss? Certainly. After all, you can't be expected to live your life without ever having another piece of chocolate or another candy cane or another toasted marshmallow around the campfire. The trick, as always, is to approach the candy shelves in your supermarket with awareness of the choices. And the key to Picture-Perfect candy choices is the consistency of the candy itself—that is, whether it's hard or soft.

Simply put, the better choice among candy options is the hard-candy choice. Here's why. You are probably not surprised to learn that jelly beans, marshmallows,

## Picture This

| 1 package (4 cookies) SnackWell's reduced-fat cookies 200 calories | = | 10 butterscotch candies 200 calories |
|---|---|---|

gummy bears, licorice, or other soft, chewy candies contain virtually no fat. Yet their calorie counts are about 100 calories per ounce, and 1 ounce of soft, chewy candies isn't very satisfying. In fact, consider the times you've scooped up a handful of jelly beans without even thinking about it. That unthinking handful is about ½ cup, the equivalent of some 400 calories.

Higher-fat candies, like chocolate, have even higher calorie counts: 120 to 160 calories per ounce. For example, a handful of M&M's (you know how easy they are to eat) contains about 520 calories.

Ounce for ounce, neither the high-fat nor the low-fat candies are calorie bargains. So why does that make hard candies a better choice for weight loss? The answer has more to do with the mind-body connection than with calories per ounce. Calorically, for the 400 calories in the handful of jelly beans, you could have 20 butterscotch candies or, if chocolate is your thing, 20 Hershey's TasteTations or eight entire Tootsie Pops. The point, however, is that it's highly unlikely that you could eat 20 butterscotch candies or 20 Taste-Tations or eight Tootsie Pops at one time. Unlike the soft candies that you chew and swallow, you suck on sour balls, lollipops, candy canes, butterscotch candies, and the like. The result is that they spend more time in your mouth, which means that your brain gets the "satisfaction message" longer. By the time the sugar has been absorbed into your bloodstream and has registered in your brain, you've had enough.

With jelly beans, for example, it's yum and they're gone—and you've just added 400 calories. With a Tootsie Pop, it's yum, yum, yum, yum, yum, at one-eighth the calorie count. The distinction may seem subtle, but it's one that can really add up—or subtract down—in terms of calories.

So as you approach the candy section in your supermarket, keep in mind the three words that all begin with hard Cs: Candy consistency counts. Hard Cs = hard candies, the better choice for Picture-Perfect Weight Loss.

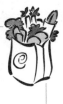

## RECOMMENDED
### Candy

❏ Tootsie Pops, Hershey's TasteTations, Werther's Originals butterscotch, or any other kind of hard candy

## Nutrition Bars

These have become all the rage lately, and in truth, they've come a long way since they first appeared some years ago. The early bars were either high-calorie candies in wrapping promising athletic prowess and good health in a single package or low-fat, high-carb bars with little nutritional value. Today's nutrition bars do indeed contain protein, fiber, vitamins, and minerals, and many of them even have reduced fat and calorie contents.

Among the more nutritious, least caloric of today's nutrition bars are Balance Bar and Luna bar. At 180 to 200 calories per bar, they're preferable, calorically speaking, to the average candy bar. That makes these nutrition bars a good potential alternative to the traditional calorie-filled, fat-soaked candy bars we've all loved since childhood: Snickers, Mars Bars, Cadbury's products, and the like.

But . . . there's always a "but," of course; in the case of nutrition bars, the "but" is all the good things I've

**Picture This**

| 1 Balance bar 200 calories | = | 10 butterscotch candies 200 calories |
|---|---|---|

## Picture This

| 1 Met-Rx bar | | 11 licorice sticks |
|---|---|---|
| 340 calories | = | 340 calories |

just said about them. Precisely because they can be nutritious and lower in calories than candy bars, nutrition bars become awfully easy to rationalize. When you feel yourself growing sluggish at 4:00 in the afternoon, you can pump yourself up with virtue if you eschew the Mars Bar in the office vending machine and instead buy the PowerBar. Of course, if you're really pressed for time or if you really need an energy hit or if the nutrition bar is absolutely your only choice, making it your afternoon pick-me-up is fine. But if you find yourself making it your afternoon pick-me-up every day or even two or three times a week, it may be time to look for less caloric choices. (The higher-calorie nutrition bars like Atkins Diet Advantage, Ultimate Locarb Bar, Met-Rx, and Pure Protein don't even bear thinking about in terms of healthy weight loss.)

Need a rule of thumb? Try the Phyllis Formula, suggested by our chief staff nutritionist, Phyllis Roxland: If you wouldn't normally buy a candy bar, think twice about spending the calories on a nutrition bar. Yes, it has nutrients that the candy bar lacks, but it still has calories. For example, it might have 100 fewer calories than the chocolate bar but 200 more than some other snacks.

Again, nutrition bars are okay when you're in dire straits every now and again, but be aware that they pack a heavy load of calories along with all that advertised nutritional power.

## RECOMMENDED
### Nutrition Bars

❏ Almost all nutrition bars have some redeeming nutritional value, but they can become a habit; so think hard about getting your nutrition elsewhere, and when you have a sweet attack, try something on the Anytime List

## Frozen Desserts

They're all right there alongside the chart-busting ice creams and frozen cakes and pies: rows of low-fat, low-calorie fudge bars, fruit bars, and other treats. But choose carefully. Not every frozen dessert advertised as "light" really lives up to the name.

For example, you would think that Weight Watchers Smart Ones products would all be pretty low in calories, but a number of these products—the ice cream sandwiches, for example—can go as high as 150 calories per bar. On the other hand, Smart Ones

## Picture This

| 1 pint low-fat ice cream 800 calories | = | 2 pints fat-free frozen yogurt 800 calories | = | 26 Tofutti Chocolate Fudge Treats 800 calories |
|---|---|---|---|---|

Berries and Cream bars, Orange Vanilla Treats, and Chocolate Mousse bars are only 40 calories per bar.

Other good fudge-bar choices are No Sugar Added Fudgsicles at 45 calories each, and Tofutti Chocolate Fudge Treats, Dolly Madison Slender Treat Chocolate Mousse bars, and Yoplait Chocolate Mousse Fudge bars, all 30 calories each.

Among fruit bars, look for Welch's sugar-free, Tropicana sugar-free, or Dole No Sugar Added at 25 calories each. At slightly higher calorie counts are frozen fruit bars that come in a great range of flavors. Try Yoplait's double fruit smoothies nonfat frozen yogurt bars at 45 calories or Häagen-Dazs fat-free chocolate sorbet bars at 80 calories or sorbet-and-yogurt bars at 90 calories. Or check out the many unusual flavors from FrozFruit—watermelon, cantaloupe, lemon, lime, strawberry—also with 90 or fewer calories; but watch out for some brands of banana or coconut, which can clock in at up to 150 calories.

Looking for pint-size nonfat frozen desserts? Shoot

for products with calorie counts under 450 per pint. Some go as low as 240 calories per pint, whether yogurt, nondairy dessert, sorbet, or Italian ice. Check out products by Häagen-Dazs, Edy's, and Seattle. Watch out for the low-fat ice creams from Mattus's, Steve's, and others: Some can go as high as 800 calories per pint!

If you don't like or can't find fat-free frozen desserts, another option is low-fat ice cream with 2 or fewer grams of fat per serving from the likes of Healthy Choice. Offered in many flavors, these are a tasty alternative to the real thing.

RECOMMENDED
**Frozen Desserts**

❏ Fudge bars: No Sugar Added Fudgsicles, Tofutti Chocolate Fudge Treats, Dolly Madison Slender Treat Chocolate Mousse, Yoplait Chocolate Mousse, Weight Watchers Smart Ones Chocolate Mousse

❏ Fruit bars: Welch's, Tropicana, or Dole No Sugar Added frozen fruit bars; Häagen-Dazs sorbet bars, FrozFruit bars

❏ Other: Weight Watchers Smart Ones Berries and Cream bar, Weight Watchers Smart Ones Orange Vanilla Treat, nonfat frozen dessert products by Häagen-Dazs, Edy's, Seattle

FROZEN DESSERTS

## Protein Foods

Think of protein foods, and you think of animal foods. Eggs, dairy products, meat, and poultry constitute the typical protein foods in the traditional American diet. Eggs for breakfast, a turkey sandwich for lunch, steak for dinner: It's how many Americans still get their protein, although millions more, worried about cholesterol, have certainly cut back on their intakes of eggs and fatty meat.

From the Picture-Perfect Weight Loss vantage, there are two important points to be made about meat, poultry, and dairy. First, all contain substances that can potentially increase your risk for cancer, heart disease, osteoporosis, diabetes, kidney disease, and a host of other ailments. Second, many of these foods tend to be high in calories and saturated fat—the bad kind.

On the other hand, many people simply cannot imagine a diet without these particular protein foods. We're not asking you to dismiss them entirely, but we do hope you will use them sparingly. The choice is yours.

One trick to reduce your intake of these protein foods is to flip the traditional ratio of main meat dish and side vegetable dish at dinner. Make the vegetables and salad the real entrée, and let the meat be just incidental—for the taste of it. Another trick is to take advantage of the low-fat versions of most meat and dairy products that are available these days. Your supermarket carries lean meat, packages of poultry with the skin removed for you, and reduced-fat and fat-free milk and cheeses. In addition, just about every manufacturer of deli foods offers poultry versions of your favorite lunchmeats—chicken franks, turkey pastrami, even turkey burgers—as well as lower-fat meat versions. All these choices save you some fat calories, but be aware that you're still taking in substances that are potentially risky to your health. In other words, fat is not the only "bad guy" in meat and poultry. And the same applies to dairy products.

Low-fat and fat-free milk, cheese, yogurt, and sour cream have all been around for a long time. Most of us are probably aware that regular dairy products are high in fat and calories. Many cheeses, for example, weigh in at 100 to 120 calories per ounce (a 1-inch cube), and most of those calories come from saturated fat. Fat-free cheese, by contrast, contains only about 40 calories per ounce but leaves a lot to be desired in the taste and consistency department. Many

PROTEIN FOODS

reduced-fat cheeses can actually be quite high in calories and fat. For example, Alpine Lace Swiss Lorraine contains 90 calories an ounce—about the same as Brie or Camembert, and with similar fat content. For these reasons, many people are starting to turn to soy cheese and other dairy alternatives.

I want to make myself clear on one point, however: Whether you usually eat the full-fat version of chicken, lamb, veal, beef, and Brie, or low-fat versions of them, you'll improve your chances for Picture-Perfect Weight Loss if you first look to other protein choices, specifically legumes, soy products, and fish. My job is to familiarize you with the healthier choices and encourage you to choose them as often as you can. Beans, soy products, and fish contain nutrients that help protect against major diseases and help keep your calorie intake down. So whenever you eat one of these protein choices, give yourself a gold star. For both weight loss and your long-term health, the more your protein comes from legumes, soy, and fish, the better. And the less protein you get from meat, poultry, and dairy, the better.

Let's turn back to these better protein choices now. We discussed one of them earlier, back in the beans aisle of our supermarket tour (see page 73).

## Focus On
### Soy

The FDA concluded that eating a small amount of soy protein per day within the context of a healthy diet can actually help reduce the risk of heart disease. The recommended amount? A mere 25 grams, or just under an ounce. The context? Your entire diet should be low in saturated fat and cholesterol.

As a result of the ruling, any food that contains at least 6.25 grams of soy protein per serving will be allowed to claim that it may help reduce the risk of heart disease. Keep in mind that substituting soy products for animal-protein foods (meat, poultry, dairy) can also reduce your risk of cancer, osteoporosis, diabetes, and kidney disease.

Beans, like all common legumes, including peas, lentils, and chickpeas, are excellent sources of protein, are rich in other nutrients, and tend to be low in calories. These are solid, right-from-the-earth vegetables that can be used in a variety of dishes and a variety of meals. Eat legumes to your heart's desire. Be assured that you're also taking in good-quality protein as you do so.

Two other excellent sources are soybeans, a very versatile vegetable that is also technically a legume, and seafood, the only animal protein with redeeming value. Let's take them one at a time.

PROTEIN FOODS

## Picture This

| 1 4-ounce beef burger 360 calories | = | 4 veggie burgers 360 calories |

Soy is a food you're probably familiar with if you've ever eaten in a Chinese or Japanese restaurant (and who hasn't?). The Japanese, in fact, eat more soy products than any other population. They also have longer life expectancies and less occurrence of heart disease, osteoporosis, and many cancers than Americans do, by far. Yet soy products are only now coming into the American mainstream and American supermarkets.

Boiled, salted green soybeans, or *edamame*, are now found in supermarkets, available both fresh and frozen. Use them in salads, as a snack, or as a side dish. In addition, supermarkets carry tofu, also known as bean curd, in the produce section. It comes in four gradations of consistency: silken, soft, firm, and extra-firm. The silken and soft work best blended into cream soups or as replacements for cream, yogurt, and other dairy products in salad dressings, dips, or shakes. The firm and extra-firm are used diced or sliced in stir-fry dishes, on the grill, or in soups.

The important thing to know about cooking with tofu is that it absorbs the flavor of whatever it's cooked with. If you've ever eaten Szechuan-style or Hunan-style bean curd from a Chinese restaurant, you know what that means. It's a dream way to take in lots of protein and disease-fighting phytochemicals—if you don't mind the top of your head coming off from the heat of the spices!

Soy also serves as a meat replacement in a range of prepared foods—an ever-widening range, as a matter of fact. Whereas at one time you could find only the occasional soy-based burger, today you can choose from an array of breakfast, lunch, and snack meat substitutes. Since the taste has improved as well, soy products today offer a nutritional blockbuster at a low calorie count—an excellent choice for Picture-Perfect Weight Loss.

Soy appears on the ingredient list as *isolated soy protein*, *textured soy protein*, *soy protein concentrate*, or *tofu*. Among burgers, look for those by Gardenburger and Boca Burger. Gardenburger's offering is 90 calories for a 2½-ounce veggie medley burger, while the Boca Burger entry is 80 calories for 2½ ounces.

Boca as well as Yves also offer a line of breakfast sausages. Boca's breakfast links are 90 calories for two

# Focus On
## Nonmeat Burgers and Franks

Both poultry-based and vegetable-based burgers and franks offer calorie advantages over the regular meat versions. But how do they stack up against one another? Zoom in here.

## Burgers

|  | Gardenburger LifeBurger (Soy Product) | Turkey Burger |
| --- | --- | --- |
| Portion size | 3 oz/85.0 g | 3 oz/82.0 g |
| Calories | 100 | 193 |
| Fat | 0 g | 10.7 g |
| Saturated fat | 0 g | 2.7 g |
| Fiber | 6.0 g | 0 g |
| Protein | 16.0 g | 22.1 g |
| Cholesterol | 0 mg | 83.6 mg |

## Franks

|  | Lightlife Smart Dog (Soy Product) | Chicken Frank |
| --- | --- | --- |
| Portion size | 42.0 g | 45.0 g |
| Calories | 45 | 116.0 |
| Fat | 0 g | 8.8 g |
| Saturated fat | 0 g | 2.5 g |
| Fiber | 0 g | 0 g |
| Protein | 9.0 g | 5.8 g |
| Cholesterol | 0 mg | 45.0 mg |

Beyond the numbers, however, choosing the veggie soy products offers an added bonus—all those plant substances, called phytochemicals, that actually decrease your risk of cancer, heart disease, osteoporosis, and other diseases.

## Picture This

| 6½-ounce package beef sausages 805 calories | = | 3 packages veggie breakfast links 805 calories |
|---|---|---|

links; its breakfast patties are 70 calories per patty. Yves veggie breakfast links weigh in at 32 calories per link.

Yves, Lightlife, and other manufacturers also offer a range of sandwich "meats," everything from ham to bologna, from Italian pepperoni to Canadian bacon. Lightlife Gimme Lean! products include a meatless sausage and a meatless ground "meat" at 70 calories for 2 ounces. Yves veggie ground round, at 60 calories for 2 ounces, is great for chili, Sloppy Joes, or tacos. Lightlife also offers a Smart Deli range that includes bologna, ham, and hot dogs. Many people say these items are better when they're spiced up with condiments or as the "meat" component of other dishes. Either on their own or as part of other dishes, however, these soy products are a great choice for nutrition and Picture-Perfect Weight Loss.

The third great source of protein is seafood,* which offers a maximum of nutrients for a minimum

*Be aware that the government recently suggested limiting intake of swordfish, shark, tile, and king mackerel because of high mercury levels and suggested that pregnant women totally avoid swordfish.

## Focus On
### Fish Tales

How do you know a good fresh fish when you see one? It should be shiny and firm enough to spring back when pressed lightly, with clear and bulging eyes. It should smell like the sea, not like fish.

As for cooking fish, the secrets are to use high heat and to stop cooking when the flesh is opaque and flakes when tested. Use the inedible parts like heads and bones—no innards—to create stock. Refrigerate leftover fish immediately; it will stay good in the refrigerator for 2 to 3 days.

of calories. Many fish are also excellent sources of the omega-3 fatty acids that are so essential to general health and as disease-fighters. What kind of seafood should you choose? Any kind, any type, any way it's sold, just about any way it's prepared (except fried).

Start at the fresh-fish counter. Throughout the year, it offers a changing choice of tastes and textures. Buy what's fresh this week and try it out. Nothing could be better for your health or your figure.

Many supermarkets also cut and prepackage fresh fish, sometimes flavoring the cut with pepper or other condiments. Eat up, but beware of prepared fish dishes with additional ingredients, especially stuffed fish, as these concoctions may contain unnecessary calories for very little taste gain.

Lots of people wonder about so-called imitation crabmeat. This is typically a little bit of real crabmeat with a lot of another fish, usually pollock. It's perfectly healthy, and very much tastes like crabmeat. In terms of nutrition and weight loss, this is a case where the imitation is just about as good as the real thing.

In many supermarkets, the smoked-fish counter is not far from the fresh-fish counter. The smoking process is, of course, aimed at preservation—and taste. So enjoy your favorite smoked fish as often as you can, whether it's "belly" lox or sablefish or sturgeon or whitefish or smoked salmon from Ireland, Scotland, Scandinavia, Nova Scotia, or the American Northwest.

Just as nutritious and low calorie as fresh and smoked fish is the canned fish you find in profusion on the shelves of your supermarket. Some canned fish—tuna, in particular—comes packed in either ' water or oil. The oil is typically canola oil, although Progresso packs its tuna in olive oil. Both oil-packed versions are healthy, and the only difference between them is taste—and the higher price of the olive oil version, especially the *virgin* olive oil version. But whether olive or canola, the oil-packed tunas are far higher in calories than tuna packed in water. The latter, therefore, is a preferable choice for Picture-Perfect Weight Loss. (You may also see some tuna in water labeled as *salt-free*; this makes no difference one way or the other to your weight-loss program, although your doctor may have restricted your salt use for other reasons.)

Apart from that caveat, indulge yourself. Sardines, kippers, clams, shrimp, crab, mackerel fillets, and anchovies all come in cans, and all are excellent choices as a main dish, in salads, and as a snack or side dish. You can also find smoked oysters, smoked clams, and smoked mussels in cans, often marketed as delicacies. They add variety to the range of tastes and, like all fish, are excellent protein choices.

Finally, don't neglect frozen fish, which offers a special level of convenience. Take the example of Contessa brand cooked shrimp. Stack a few of these packages in your freezer; then, whenever you hanker for a shrimp cocktail, just open one, run cold water over the shrimp for 10 minutes, add cocktail sauce, and you're done. At 30 calories per

PROTEIN FOODS

ounce, with a couple of tablespoons of cocktail sauce weighing in at 22 calories, it's a filling, healthful, very low calorie dish.

Or throw the defrosted shrimp into a salad. Serve them on a platter of cooked vegetables. The possibilities are almost endless. The same goes for the frozen tuna or salmon burgers in your supermarket's freezer chest. Defrost and broil one, or marinate it in a light salad dressing or soy sauce, then grill or bake, and you have a low-calorie, healthy, easy main dish.

My one caveat about frozen fish is prepared seafood dishes, which *can* be very high in calories. Contessa shrimp scampi, for example, weighs in at 430 calories for 4 ounces. Not all prepared seafoods are calorically off the charts. A serving of stuffed clams, at 130 calories, is hefty enough to serve as an entrée, while Plumpy brand's mussels in mild tomato sauce are only 100 calories per serving, and Chesapeake Bay crab cakes, very low fat, are an okay 60 calories per crab cake. But when a package of frozen fish boasts a name or photo referring to something other than just fish, check the label carefully. There's plenty of choice. Instead of the 4 ounces of shrimp scampi for 430 calories, for example, try Icy Bay's langostinos. At 4 ounces with

60 calories, they're a far better choice for Picture-Perfect Weight Loss.

### Prote n Foods

❑ Legumes: beans, peas, lentils, chickpeas
❑ Soy products: bean curd/tofu, meat-replacement
   products by Boca, Gardenburger, Yves, Lightlife
❑ Seafood: fresh (do not fry!), smoked, canned, frozen

## Alcoholic Beverages

Whether o- not your supermarket stocks alcoholic beverages depends on which state you live in. In some states, only beer is available in supermarke-s; other state laws aLow beer and wine to be sold; and in some places, supermarkets carry a full line of alcohol. Finally, certain states allow alcohol to be solc only in specialized ɔeer or liquor stores or in "state stores."

For the weight conscious, wherever yoɯ find alcoholic beverages, it's a good idea to choose thoughtfully and cautiously. Unless you're using wine as a cooking ingredient—in which case you're using very little, most of which will be cooked off—alcoholic beverages can be troublesome.

For one thing, they tend to have a fairly high

calorie count. In general, alcoholic drinks contain 7 calories per gram. How does that translate into actual drinks? Six ounces of wine or champagne, to take one example, weighs in at about 130 calories. A 12-ounce can of beer costs approximately 145 calories; the count is 160 to 200 if it's dark beer, 96 to 110 for lite beer. Hard liquor is clocked at 60 to 90 calories per ounce, depending on the proof, and most poured drinks have 2 ounces (probably more if you pour them yourself). Add in the calories of whatever you're mixing in to create the cocktail, and your evening drink could be costing you 240 calories or more. At holiday time, a single eggnog, with alcohol, sugar, and saturated fat, could run from 400 to 650 calories!

The problem is, it's difficult to have just one single drink, and the more you have, the more you tend to eat. Alcohol is a real spur to appetite. That's what is truly troublesome about an evening cocktail or wine with dinner or a beer while you're watching the ball game.

This is physiological fact, not moral preaching. Alcohol increases appetite by lowering your blood sugar, triggering hunger. It also depresses your central nervous system—specifically, those areas that act as restraints on behavior. The double-whammy result is that you both feel hungry and lose your inhibitions. You're simply more willing to eat whatever's around. And "whatever's around" when people are drinking tends to be high-calorie munchies at a cocktail party or a rich meal at a restaurant or a lavish dessert at a dinner party—the sorts of foods you would not ordinarily buy or prepare for yourself.

This does not mean that I think you should give up alcohol if it's something you enjoy. In moderation, wine, beer, and spirits belong to the great variety of tastes and textures that are part of eating and part of life. Again, the issue is awareness, and the problem with alcohol is remaining aware of what you're taking in as you enjoy that ice-cold martini or that lovely glass of Merlot or that chilled beer after a long day at work.

Here's the tip I give my patients: Make the first drink of the evening water or club soda on the rocks, with lemon or lime, if you like. Why? Because the first drink always seems to go down quickly, whether it's a white-wine spritzer or a double vodka Collins or a glass of water. That being the case, make it a glass of water or diet beverage. Sip it slowly if you can, or at least sip at the same rate that those around you are downing their glasses of wine or vodka or beer. Wait for the second drink before you order an alcoholic beverage. You'll save not only the calories of the alcohol but also the calories of that creamy dip you held out against or that high-fat dish you decided not to order from the menu or that basket of bread you didn't eat while you waited for your meal or that dessert you were able to say no to. It's a lot to gain by giving up just one drink.

## Chapter 5

# FOOD SABOTEURS

*S*aboteur. It even sounds ominous. Sinister. Vaguely dangerous.

Saboteurs deal in disguise. They are not what they seem. They say one thing but mean another. *The American Heritage Dictionary of the English Language, Third Edition* says that saboteurs practice treachery and secrecy "to defeat or hinder a cause or endeavor."

That's exactly what food saboteurs do. They look benign enough. Sometimes, they even promise to be weight-control helpers; they hint that they can actually assist us in our weight-loss endeavor. "Fat-free!" they proclaim. Or "Reduced sugar!" Or "No cholesterol!" Or "All-natural ingredients!" Lulled by these claims, we give ourselves permission to indulge in these foods, only to find that we have rationalized overeating them. If a cookie is sugar-free, why not indulge? If the muffin is fat-free, why not have a big one for breakfast? If the pretzels are low salt and therefore "good for us," we may as well have a handful, especially since it will take at least a handful to be satisfied by the low-salt taste.

The result? Instead of helping us lose weight, food saboteurs may actually lead to our putting on more weight.

## Let the Buyer Beware

What's so treacherous about these foods? What makes them saboteurs? The answer is simple: Tempted by the food and beguiled by its elusive label lingo, we let down our Food Awareness guard.

Once that happens, we forget or fail to consider that these foods, for the most part, are packed with calories. Not only that, these are empty calories that lack nutritional benefits. There's no bargain here—no added nutritional value to compensate for a high calorie count. On the contrary.

That's why food saboteurs are the only foods you should avoid for Picture-Perfect Weight Loss. They're not bad foods. Remember, *there are no bad foods*. But they are bad choices for people trying to maintain awareness about weight control.

And they are everywhere. The staff nutritionists at my weight-loss clinic in New York divide the food saboteurs into two main categories, the so-called *haves*

## Picture This

| 1 6-ounce bag vegetable chips 840 calories | = | 21 pretzel rods 840 calories |
|---|---|---|

and the *have-nots*. The *haves* are foods that claim a re-deeming nutritional benefit: "honey sweetened" rather than "sugar sweetened," or chips made from taro, not potatoes. Such foods lull us with their promise to add healthfulness, despite the calories. The *have-nots*, by contrast, boast the ingredients they do *not* contain, for instance, no fat, no sugar, no salt, no cholesterol. They lull us with their promise of the danger we're escaping.

It's a hoax on both counts. For both the haves and the have-nots can sabotage your weight-loss efforts and undermine the results.

## The So-Called Haves: Doing What Comes Naturally?

Remember those granola and muesli cereals we looked at on our supermarket tour in chapter 4, the ones containing nuts, coconut, seeds, dried fruit, and the like? The ones claiming—rightly—to be filled with nutritious ingredients? They're a perfect example of the haves category of food saboteur. So healthy. So delicious. So why not have a really big bowl of them in the morning? Why not reach for them when you crave a sweet snack—just pull a few handfuls out of the box and munch away?

There's a reason why not. The calorie counts of these cereals are stratospheric.

There's another good name for the saboteur haves. I refer to them as the *healthy naturals*. They include the candy bar made with carob instead of chocolate, the pretzels covered in yogurt rather than white chocolate, the chips made from taro or beets or some vegetable other than potatoes, the cookie sweetened with honey instead of sugar.

## Focus On
### Calcium

Where, besides dairy products, can you get the calcium that is so needed by everyone, especially women over 50? Among Picture-Perfect Weight Loss choices, here's where, in descending order from highest to lowest amounts: sardines with bones, oranges, soy milk, collard greens, salmon, turnip or beet greens, oatmeal, fortified cereal, baked beans, soybeans, tofu, kale, broccoli, and white beans.

## Picture This

| 1 package (3 ounces) yogurt-covered raisins 360 calories | = | 40 dried apricot halves 360 calories |
|---|---|---|

At least, we tell ourselves, these are not empty-calorie foods. At least we're not eating "junk." Yogurt, root vegetables, honey from bees: What could be bad?

Nothing, of course. Only there isn't much that's particularly good, either. There's no added nutritional benefit. No particular weight-loss advantage accrues because you've changed an ingredient. The honey-sweetened cookie is just as caloric as the one sweetened with sugar. The taro chip is just as caloric and just as fat filled as the potato chip. The same is true of the pretzels: Covering them with yogurt instead of white chocolate doesn't lower the calorie or fat content; it just makes you seem virtuous instead of indulgent.

You gain nothing except weight with the healthy naturals. But since you can so easily persuade yourself that there is a nutritional boon, which there isn't, you run the risk of eating more calories than if you were to stick with the real thing.

When cruising the aisles of your supermarket, apply the Phyllis Formula, devised by our chief staff nutritionist, Phyllis Roxland. We first talked about it in chapter 4, in the section on nutrition bars. Where food saboteurs are concerned, Phyllis says that you should ask yourself if you would have chosen the regular snack—the sugar-sweetened cookie or the potato chips—if you were shopping with your "regular" awareness about food and weight control. If the answer is no, that proves that the juice-sweetened cookie or taro-chip substitute is actually adding more calories to your diet—calories you would have avoided otherwise. The substitute is, in short, a way of rationalizing a food choice that you actually weren't that interested in eating in the first place.

You've worked hard to raise your Food Awareness. You're making progress, controlling your weight. You've done it all by making your own food choices. There are plenty of low-fat, low-calorie foods on the Picture-Perfect Anytime List. Fill your shopping cart with these—and beware the food saboteurs!

## The Have-Nots: Fat-Free, Sugar-Free, Cholesterol-Free

One of the worst things to happen to weight-conscious people in this country was the introduction of

## Picture This

| 1 low-fat corn muffin (6 ounces) 480 calories | = | 4 English muffins 480 calories |
| --- | --- | --- |

fat-free baked goods. Marie Antoinette saying, "Let them eat cake!" could not have provided a better introduction to what happened next: Like sinners who have been given absolution, people flocked to the supermarkets to indulge their tastes for cakes, muffins, cookies, and a range of new confections.

And the nation as a whole promptly gained weight.

Why? Because people were under the impression that only calories from fat would make them gain weight, and the "fat-free" label let them rationalize away a lot of refined-carbohydrate calories. The baked goods they now consumed *without thinking about it* were just as high in calories and as low in nutrition as they had been before the "fat-free" label was attached. People just didn't know it, or perhaps they simply convinced themselves otherwise. They had just exchanged one nutritional culprit for another, substituting refined carbs for fat. But they were still taking in just as many calories. In fact, "freed" to consume more baked goods, they were actually taking in more calories.

## The Snack Sand Trap

Snack foods are particularly dangerous have-not saboteurs. Their packages scream with boasts about all the "bad" ingredients they don't have or have in "low" or "reduced" amounts: fat, sugar, sodium, cholesterol. What these foods do have, however, are calories.

The research has made it clear.

ITEM: Two Drake's Yodels contain 280 calories. Two Drake's Reduced-Fat Yodels contain 290 calories.

ITEM: Two tablespoons of Jif peanut butter contain 190 calories. The number of calories in 2 tablespoons of Jif's reduced-fat version? Exactly the same: 190.

ITEM: Five Nabisco Premium Saltines contain 60 calories. Five Nabisco fat-free Premium Saltines also contain 60 calories.

The danger is that you will eat more of the fat-free version, both because it will take more to satisfy the palate and because the fat-free label persuades you that it is okay to eat more.

My personal favorite among these claims is the

"No Cholesterol!" assertion plastered all over packages of potato chips and frozen french fries. True, these foods have no cholesterol. No food that comes from a plant has cholesterol. What both foods do have, however, is a whopping amount of fats—and bad fats, at that, including the dreaded trans fat, a major enemy of heart health.

If you have a hankering for a salty snack, try a dill pickle, with between 5 and 20 calories in a giant one. If you crave something sweet and baked, how about an English muffin with jam for under 200 calories?

In any event, it's best to keep these have-not saboteurs out of your market basket. Need a rule of thumb? Again, rely on the Phyllis Formula. Would I choose this bag of potato chips if it weren't labeled "cholesterol-free"? If the answer is no, move on. Find something from the Picture-Perfect Anytime List on page 15 instead.

## Classic Food Saboteurs: Beware!

### *The So-Called Haves/Healthy Naturals:*

- Granola, trail mix
- Vegetable chips
- Carob candies, cookies

- Yogurt-covered pretzels or raisins
- Naturally sweetened or fruit-juice-sweetened cakes, cookies, beverages

### The Have-Nots

- Fat-free and low-fat cakes, cookies, muffins, chips, pretzels, crackers
- Sugar-free or dietetic candy, cookies, cakes
- Salt-free or cholesterol-free snack foods like chips, crackers, popcorn, pretzels

# Sugar Replacements

Do you want a sugar replacement? Or, do you want to know what you're ingesting when the food you eat contains a sugar replacement? Check out the facts on sugar substitutes in the table that follows.

The benchmark against which to measure these replacements is, of course, sugar itself—plain old table sugar, the stuff you sprinkle over your morning cereal or add to your coffee. Its official name is sucrose, and it contains 4 calories per gram (4 cal/g). The table shows just how the replacements measure up.

| Replacement | Trade/Other Names | Description/Use | Cal/g |
|---|---|---|---|
| Sorbitol | None | 50%–70% as sweet as sugar; excessive amounts (more than 20 g) may act as a laxative in some people | 2.6 |
| Mannitol | None | 50%–70% as sweet as sugar; excessive amounts (more than 20 g) may act as a laxative in some people | 1.6 |
| Xylitol | None | As sweet as sugar | 2.4 |
| Erythritol | None | 70% as sweet as sugar | 0.2 |
| Lactitol | None | 30%–40% as sweet as sugar; used as a bulking agent | 2.0 |
| Isomalt | None | 45%–65% as sweet as sugar | 2.0 |

*(continued)*

| Replacement | Trade/Other Names | Description/Use | Cal/g |
|---|---|---|---|
| Maltitol | None | 90% as sweet as sugar | 3.0 |
| Hydrogenated starch hydrolysates | HSH; maltitol syrup | 25%–50% as sweet as sugar | 3.0 |
| Saccharin | Sweet 'N Low | 200%–700% sweeter than sugar; noncariogenic; produces no glycemic response—i.e., no increase in blood sugar; synergizes the sweetening power of caloric and noncaloric sweeteners; the sweetening effect is not diminished by heating | 0 |
| Aspartame | NutraSweet; Equal | 160%–220% sweeter than sugar; noncariogenic; produces limited glycemic response; new forms can increase its sweetening effect in cooking and baking | 4* |
| Acesulfame-K | Sunett | 200% sweeter than sugar; noncariogenic; produces no glycemic response; sweetening effect not diminished by heating; can synergize the sweetening power of other caloric and noncaloric sweeteners | 0 |
| Sucralose | Splenda | 600% sweeter than sugar; noncariogenic; produces no glycemic response; sweetening effect is not diminished by heating | 0 |

*Provides limited calories to food products because of its sweetening power—that is, because the sweetener is highly concentrated, the tendency is to use it in small amounts.

# FAT REPLACEMENTS

Just as sugar replacements provide a sweet taste, fat replacements give food the flavor or consistency of fat without the calories. For anyone trying to cut down on his or her intake of fat, for health or any other reasons, the table that follows shows the calorie counts of these replacements in calories per gram (cal/g). For comparison, 1 gram of fat has a whopping 9 calories. Of course, many foods always were and always will be fat-free—angel food cake and cornflakes are two premier examples—but their calorie counts are another matter altogether. So whether a food is inherently low fat or whether it is low fat by virtue of a fat replacement, it is not necessarily a low-calorie food.

| Replacement | Trade/Other Names | Description/Use | Cal/g |
|---|---|---|---|
| Maltodextrin, corn syrup solid, hydrolyzed corn starch, modified food starch, polydextrose | Maltrin, Lycadex, Paselli Excel, Stellar | Frozen desserts, cheese, baked goods, sauces, dressings, sour cream, yogurt, breads, meats, and poultry | 1.0 when hydrated in a product |
| Pectin, carrageenan, sugar beet fiber of powder, cellulose gel, xanthan gum, guar gum | Slendid, Viscarin, Fibrex, Avicel, Pycol, Jaguar | Yogurt, sour cream, salad dressings, bakery products, frozen desserts, cheese spreads, sauces | 0–0.5 |

*(continued)*

| Replacement | Trade/Other Names | Description/Use | Cal/g |
|---|---|---|---|
| Hydrogenated starch hydrolysate, hydrogenated glucose syrup, sorbitol, maltitol, polydextrose | Lycasin, Hystar, Neosor, Litesse, Sta-Lite | Baked goods, confections, chewing gum, frozen dairy desserts, gelatins, puddings, sauces, salad dressings, meat-based products | 1.0–4.0 |
| Microparticulated egg white and milk protein, whey protein concentrate | Simplesse, K-Blazer, Lita, Dairy-Lo | Cheese, butter, mayonnaise, salad dressings, sour cream, bakery products, spreads | 1.3 |
| Caprenin | Salatrim | Chocolate and confections, cookies, crackers | 5.0 |
| Olestra | Olean | Savory snacks (like chips) and crackers | 0 |

# MY PERSONAL PICTURE-PERFECT SHOPPING LIST
## (With Dr. Shapiro's Recommendations)

### Beverages*

- ❑ Diet (or low-calorie or light) flavored drinks
- ❑ Diet sodas
- ❑ Diet iced teas
- ❑ Waters

### Cereals

- ❑ Cheerios
- ❑ Kellogg's All-Bran
- ❑ Original Shredded Wheat
- ❑ Wheaties
- ❑ Kellogg's Special K
- ❑ Kellogg's Product 19
- ❑ Whole Grain Total
- ❑ Oatmeal
- ❑ Fiber One
- ❑ Bran Flakes

## Spreads

- ❑ Real peanut butter
- ❑ Low-sugar or sugar-free jams and jellies

## Breads

- ❑ Light breads
- ❑ Whole grain regular bread or rolls

## Sauces, Condiments, and Marinades*

- ❑ Tomato sauce, ketchup, barbecue sauce
- ❑ Mustard
- ❑ Relish, chutney, salsa
- ❑ Fat-free and light salad dressing
- ❑ Soy sauce, teriyaki sauce
- ❑ Black bean sauce, miso, duck sauce, hoisin sauce

## Dips*

- ❑ Salsas
- ❑ Bean dips
- ❑ Light creamy salad dressings
- ❑ Hummus
- ❑ Baba ghannouj

## Rice and Pasta

- ❏ Whole wheat/whole grain pastas
- ❏ Brown rice
- ❏ Other whole grains: quinoa, whole wheat couscous, whole grain cornmeal, kasha, bulgur wheat, barley, millet

## Soups*

(Avoid noodle- or rice-based or cream soups high in saturated fats.)

- ❏ Lentil, split pea
- ❏ Minestrone
- ❏ Black bean
- ❏ Tomato-vegetable
- ❏ Miso, hot and sour, Chinese vegetable
- ❏ Pureed vegetable soups: carrot, butternut squash, etc.

## Frozen Meals

- ❏ Low-calorie frozen breakfast foods
- ❏ Low-calorie, vegetable-focused frozen meals

## Dressings and Oils*

- ❑ Light ready-made dressings
- ❑ Flavored vinegars
- ❑ Unsaturated oils (in moderation)

## Beans

- ❑ Dried
- ❑ Canned
- ❑ Health Valley canned bean-chili combinations
- ❑ Low-fat or fat-free refried beans

## Produce and Fresh Food*

All highly recommended—write your favorites here.

- ❑ _____
- ❑ _____
- ❑ _____
- ❑ _____
- ❑ _____
- ❑ _____

## Snacks*

Starchy, crunchy snacks (best eaten in moderation)
- ❏ Pretzel rods
- ❏ Lite popcorn
- ❏ Rice cakes
- ❏ Whole grain/high-fiber crackers or flat breads
- ❏ Reduced-fat corn or potato chips

## Candy*

- ❏ Tootsie Pops
- ❏ Hershey's TasteTations
- ❏ Werther's Originals
- ❏ Other hard candy
- ❏ Gum

## Nutrition Bars

Think hard about this choice.
- ❏ Balance Bar
- ❏ Luna bar

## Frozen Desserts*

### *Fudge Bars*

- ❏ Sugar-free Fudgsicles
- ❏ Tofutti Chocolate Fudge Treats
- ❏ Dolly Madison Slender Treat Chocolate Mousse
- ❏ Yoplait Chocolate Mousse
- ❏ Weight Watchers Smart Ones Chocolate Mousse

### *Fruit Bars*

- ❏ Welch's No-Sugar-Added Fruit Juice Bars
- ❏ Tropicana sugar-free popsicles
- ❏ Häagen-Dazs sorbet or yogurt bars
- ❏ FrozFruit bars
- ❏ Sugar-free popsicles

### *Other*

- ❏ Weight Watchers Smart Ones Berries and Cream bar
- ❏ Weight Watchers Smart Ones Orange Vanilla Treat
- ❏ Nonfat frozen dessert products by Häagen-Dazs, Edy's, Seattle
- ❏ Sugar-free Creamsicles

# Protein Foods

### Legumes

- ❑ Beans
- ❑ Peas
- ❑ Lentils
- ❑ Chickpeas

### Soy Products

- ❑ Bean curd/tofu
- ❑ Meat–replacement products by Boca, Gardenburger, Yves, Lightlife

### Seafood*

- ❑ Fresh
- ❑ Smoked
- ❑ Canned
- ❑ Frozen

*Be aware that the government recently suggested limiting intake of swordfish, shark, tile, and king mackerel because of high mercury levels and suggested that pregnant women totally avoid swordfish.

## Alcoholic Beverages

Buy—and drink—in moderation.

- ❑ Wine/champagne
- ❑ Light beer

*\*For My Picture-Perfect Anytime List: foods that should fill up my pantry, refrigerator, and freezer so I can reach for them anytime when I want a snack or am planning a meal.*

# CALORIE COUNTER

This handy calorie counter contains foods commonly found on supermarket shelves. Pay attention to portion information on this list and always read the labels on the packages of food you are considering. Different brands of food often have different calorie counts.

Some of the foods on this list are recommended in the book; others are not. It is for quick reference only, and is not a substitute or short version of the material in this book. In fact, while calories are important, there are sometimes good reasons for choosing a higher-calorie food. For my recommendations and full explanation of how to make the best choices for Picture-Perfect Weight Loss, see the body of this book.

## Alcoholic Beverages

| Serving Size | Item | Calories |
|---|---|---|
| 1½ oz | Distilled Liquor | 100 |
| 12 oz | Light Beer | 100 |
| 6 oz | White Wine | 120 |
| 6 oz | Red Wine | 125 |
| 12 oz | Wine Spritzer | 140 |
| 12 oz | Beer | 145 |

*(continued)*

## Alcoholic Beverages—continued

| Serving Size | Item | Calories |
|---|---|---|
| 12 oz | Dark Beer | 160 |
| 1 (average) | Screwdriver | 175 |
| 6 oz | Dessert Wine | 220 |
| 6 oz | Wine Cooler | 230 |
| 1 (average) | Piña Colada | 260 |
| 1 (average) | Martini | 500 |

## Beans

| Serving Size | Item | Calories |
|---|---|---|
| ½ cup | Green and Yellow Wax Beans | 20 |
| ½ cup | Green Peas | 60 |
| ½ cup | Eden Soybeans, Canned | 90 |
| ½ cup | Black-Eyed Peas | 100 |
| ½ cup | Progresso Cannellini Beans, Canned | 100 |
| ½ cup | Healthy Valley Fat-Free Baked Beans | 110 |
| ½ cup | Kidney Beans | 110 |
| ½ cup | Lima Beans | 110 |
| ½ cup | Old El Paso Pinto Beans, Canned | 110 |
| ½ cup | Progresso Black Beans, Canned | 110 |
| ½ cup | Lentils | 115 |
| ½ cup | Split Peas | 115 |
| ½ cup | Chickpeas | 120 |
| ½ cup | Low-Fat Refried Beans | 140 |
| ½ cup | B&M Baked Beans | 170 |

# Beverages

| Serving Size | Item | Calories |
|---|---|---|
| 12 oz | Club Soda | 0 |
| 8 oz | Diet Raspberry Snapple Ice Tea | 0 |
| 12 oz | Diet Sunkist Orange | 0 |
| 8 oz | Diet Natural Lemon Nestea | 2 |
| 12 oz | Diet Rite | 2 |
| 8 oz | Crystal Light | 5 |
| 6 oz | Swiss Miss Diet and Fat-Free Cocoa | 50 |
| 1 serving | Alba Milkshake | 70 |
| 1 serving | Weight Watchers Milkshake | 80 |
| 12 oz | Regular Soda | 150 |
| 12 oz | Chocolate Milkshake | 430 |

# Breads

| Serving Size | Item | Calories |
|---|---|---|
| 1 slice | Arnold's Light Bread | 40 |
| 1 slice | Low-Calorie Wheat Bread | 45 |
| 1 slice | Pepperidge Farm Light Style | 45 |
| 1 slice | Roman Meal | 65 |
| 1 slice | Whole Wheat Bread | 70 |
| 1 slice | French Bread | 80 |
| 1 slice | Pepperidge Farm Cinnamon Swirl Bread | 80 |
| 1 slice | Bran'ola Original | 90 |
| 1 slice | Pepperidge Farm Nine Grain | 90 |

*(continued)*

## Breads—continued

| Serving Size | Item | Calories |
|---|---|---|
| 1 average | Hamburger Roll | 125 |
| 1 | English Muffin | 135 |
| 1 | Pepperidge Farm Multigrain Roll | 150 |
| 1 (6½ inch) | Pita | 165 |
| 1 medium (2 oz) | Croissant | 230 |
| 1 (3½ oz) | Flaky Biscuit | 360 |
| 1 (3½ oz) | Garlic Bread | 360 |
| 1 (5 oz) | Bagel | 400 |

## Candy

| Serving Size | Item | Calories |
|---|---|---|
| 5 | Hershey's TasteTations | 100 |
| 5 | Lifesavers | 100 |
| 5 | Starburst Fruit Chews | 100 |
| 2 | Tootsie Pops | 100 |
| 5 | Werther's Original Butterscotch | 100 |
| 10 | Large Jelly Beans | 105 |
| 10 | Small Gum Drops | 135 |
| 4 | Twizzlers Black Licorice | 140 |
| 1 (1½ oz) | York Peppermint Patties | 165 |
| 5 pieces | Kraft Peanut Brittle | 170 |
| 1 pack (1.69 oz) | M&M's | 235 |

## Cereals

| Serving Size | Item | Calories |
|---|---|---|
| ½ cup | Kellogg's All-Bran with Extra Fiber | 50 |
| ½ cup | Fiber One | 60 |
| 1 biscuit | Original Shredded Wheat | 80 |
| 1 cup | General Mill's Multi-Grain Cheerios | 110 |
| 1 cup | Kellogg's Product 19 | 110 |
| 1 cup | Wheaties | 110 |
| ¾ cup | Whole Grain Total | 110 |
| 1 cup | Farina | 115 |
| 1 cup | Kellogg's Special K | 115 |
| 1 cup | Cream of Wheat | 135 |
| 1 cup | Wheatena | 135 |
| 1 cup | Arrowhead Mills Oat Bran Flakes | 140 |
| 1 cup | Ralston Purina Bran Chex | 155 |
| 1 cup | Kellogg's Raisin Bran Cereal | 185 |
| ½ cup | Healthy Choice Low-Fat Granola without Raisins | 190 |
| 1 cup | General Mill's Raisin-Nut Bran | 210 |
| ½ cup | Grape-Nuts | 210 |
| ⅔ cup | Healthy Choice Low-Fat Granola with Raisins | 220 |
| ½ cup | Granola | 260 |
| 1 cup | Ralston Purina Muesli Peach Pecan | 270 |

## Dips

| Serving Size | Item | Calories |
|---|---|---|
| 2 Tbsp | Salsa | 10 |
| 2 Tbsp | Old El Paso Black Bean Dip | 25 |
| 2 Tbsp | Chi-Chi's Fiesta Cheese Dip | 40 |
| 2 Tbsp | Old El Paso Cheese 'n Salsa Dip | 40 |
| 2 Tbsp | Kraft Clam Dip | 45 |
| 2 Tbsp | Hummus | 50 |
| 2 Tbsp | Kraft French Onion Dip | 50 |
| 2 Tbsp | Breakstone's Bacon and Onion Sour Cream Dip | 60 |
| 2 Tbsp | Kraft Avocado Dip | 60 |
| 2 Tbsp | Heluva Good Pretzel Cheddar and Mustard Dip | 80 |
| 1 Tbsp | Tahini | 85 |
| 2 Tbsp | Marie's Spinach Dip | 140 |
| 2 Tbsp | Marie's Bacon Ranch Dip | 150 |

## Dressings and Oils

| Serving Size | Item | Calories |
|---|---|---|
| 2 Tbsp | Regina Red Wine Vinegar with Garlic | 0 |
| 2 Tbsp | Balsamic Vinegar | 10 |
| 2 Tbsp | Good Seasons Fat-Free Zesty Italian | 10 |
| 2 Tbsp | Seven Seas Free Red Wine Vinegar | 15 |
| 2 Tbsp | Hidden Valley Fat-Free Italian Parmesan | 20 |
| 2 Tbsp | Marie's Low-Fat Zesty Ranch | 30 |

| 2 Tbsp | Wish-Bone Just 2 Good Italian | 35 |
|---|---|---|
| 2 Tbsp | Marie's Fat-Free White Wine Vinaigrette | 40 |
| 2 Tbsp | Wish-Bone Just 2 Good Classic Caesar | 40 |
| 2 Tbsp | Maple Grove Farms of Vermont Poppyseed | 45 |
| 2 Tbsp | Good Season's Reduced-Calorie Italian | 50 |
| 2 Tbsp | Kraft Fat-Free Blue Cheese | 50 |
| 2 Tbsp | Hellmann's Citrus Splash | 90 |
| 2 Tbsp | Seven Seas Creamy Italian | 110 |
| 2 Tbsp | Wish-Bone French | 120 |
| 1 Tbsp | Oil (Vegetable, Olive, Nut, or Seed) | 125 |
| 2 Tbsp | Kraft Honey Dijon | 155 |
| 2 Tbsp | Caesar Dressing | 160 |
| 2 Tbsp | Kraft Ranch | 165 |
| 2 Tbsp | Marie's Chunky Blue Cheese | 180 |

## Frozen Desserts

| Serving Size | Item | Calories |
|---|---|---|
| 1 | Dole No Sugar Added Fruit Bar | 25 |
| 1 | Tropicana Sugar-Free Fruit Bar | 25 |
| 1 | Welch's Sugar-Free Fruit Bar | 25 |
| 1 | Dolly Madison Slender Treat Chocolate Mousse Bar | 30 |
| 1 | Tofutti Chocolate Fudge Treats | 30 |
| 1 | Yoplait Chocolate Mousse Fudge Bar | 30 |
| 1 | Weight Watchers Smart Ones Berries and Cream Bars | 40 |

*(continued)*

## Frozen Desserts—continued

| Serving Size | Item | Calories |
|---|---|---|
| 1 | No Sugar Added Fudgsicle | 45 |
| 1 | Yoplait's Nonfat Frozen Yogurt Bar | 45 |
| 1 | Häagen-Dazs Fat-Free Chocolate Sorbet Bar | 80 |
| 1 | Creamsicle | 90 |
| 1 | FrozFruit Bar | 90 |
| 1 | Häagen-Dazs Sorbet and Yogurt Bar | 90 |
| ½ cup | Edy's Fat-Free Black Cherry Vanilla Ice Cream | 100 |
| ½ cup | Healthy Choice Low-Fat Vanilla | 100 |
| 1 (6 oz) | Luigi's Strawberry Italian Ice | 110 |
| ½ cup | Healthy Choice Low-Fat Cookies and Cream | 120 |
| ½ cup | Breyer's Low-Fat Red Raspberry Frozen Yogurt | 125 |
| ½ cup | Häagen-Dazs Chocolate Chocolate Chip | 300 |
| ½ cup | Ben and Jerry's Butter Pecan Ice Cream | 310 |
| 1 | Dove Bar, Chocolate with Dark Chocolate | 330 |

## Frozen Meals
### Breakfast

| Serving Size | Item | Calories |
|---|---|---|
| 1 | Kellogg's Eggo Blueberry Pancake | 150 |
| 1 (2 oz) | Lender's Cinnamon Swirl Bagel | 150 |
| 2 | Aunt Jemima Buttermilk Pancakes | 160 |

| | | |
|---|---|---|
| 2 | Aunt Jemima Whole Grain Waffles | 160 |
| 3 | Pillsbury Harvest Wheat Pancakes | 160 |
| 2 | Krusteaz Cinnamon Swirl French Toast | 175 |
| 2 | Eggo Nutri-Grain Waffles | 190 |
| 1 | Swanson Great Starts Egg and Bacon Burrito | 250 |
| 1 | Swanson Great Starts Sausage, Egg, and Cheese Biscuit | 460 |

## Lunch/Dinner

| Serving Size | Item | Calories |
|---|---|---|
| 1 | Amy's Shepherd's Pie | 160 |
| 1 | Stouffer's Lean Cuisine Mexican Tamale Pie | 220 |
| 1 | Healthy Choice Garlic Milano Chicken | 240 |
| 1 | Stouffer's Lean Cuisine Asian Noodle Stir-Fry | 240 |
| 1 | Celentano's Low-Fat Manicotti | 250 |
| 1 | Celentano's Low-Fat Stuffed Shells | 250 |
| 1 | Healthy Choice Pasta Italiano | 250 |
| 1 | Stouffer's Lean Cuisine 3-Bean Chili | 250 |
| 1 | Celentano's Low-Fat Lasagna | 260 |
| 1 | Stouffer's Lean Cuisine Santa-Fe–Style Rice and Beans | 300 |
| 1 | Stouffer's Lean Cuisine Tofu Vegetable Lasagna | 300 |
| 1 | Stouffer's Lean Cuisine Vegetable Egg Roll | 300 |
| 1 | Tai Gourmet Vegetable Korma | 300 |
| 1 | Stouffer's Lean Cuisine Cannelloni with Vegetables | 350 |

## Nutrition Bars

| Serving Size | Item | Calories |
|---|---|---|
| 1 | Everyday (Chocolate Fudge) | 170 |
| 1 | Luna Bar (Lemon) | 180 |
| 1 | Boost (Chocolate Crunch) | 190 |
| 1 | Balance Bar (Chocolate) | 200 |
| 1 | 151 Bar (Chocolate Cappuccino) | 210 |
| 1 | Pounds Off (Chocolate Fudge) | 210 |
| 1 | Slim-Fast (Chocolate Cookie Dough) | 220 |
| 1 | Tiger Sport (Chocolate) | 230 |
| 1 | Clif Bar (Carrot Cake) | 240 |
| 1 | Pure Protein (Chocolate Deluxe) | 270 |
| 1 | Premier Protein (Yogurt Peanut Crunch) | 290 |
| 1 | Met-Rx (Fudge Brownie) | 340 |

## Produce

Fresh fruits and vegetables range from 7 calories (a cup of lettuce) to 170 calories (a baked potato) per serving. We recommend them all.

## Protein Foods

| Serving Size | Item | Calories |
|---|---|---|
| 1 slice | Galaxy's Veggie Slices (Mozzarella) | 20 |
| 3 oz | Mori-Nu Lite Tofu | 35 |
| 1 oz | Lightlife Smart Deli Stick (Pepperoni) | 45 |
| 1 | Lightlife Smart Dog | 45 |

| | | |
|---|---|---|
| 2 cakes | Chesapeake Bay Crab Cakes | 60 |
| 1 (2½ oz) | Boca Burger | 80 |
| 3 oz | Crabmeat, Steamed | 85 |
| 3 oz | Shrimp, Steamed | 85 |
| 1 (2½ oz) | Gardenburger Hamburger-Style Soy Pattie | 90 |
| 2 links | Yves Veggie Breakfast Links | 90 |
| 3 oz | Albacore Tuna Packed in Water | 105 |
| 3 oz | Haddock, Broiled or Baked | 95 |
| 1 oz | Gardenburger Life Burger | 100 |
| 1 | Morningstar Farms Garden Veggie Patties | 100 |
| 3 oz | Salmon, Smoked | 100 |
| 1 oz | Cheese, Cheddar | 110 |
| ½ cup | Kidney Beans | 110 |
| ½ cup | Lentils | 115 |
| ½ cup | Chickpeas | 120 |
| ½ cup | Split Peas | 120 |
| ½ cup | Soybeans | 125 |
| 1 cup | Soy Milk | 140 |
| 1 | Beef Hot Dog | 145 |
| 3 oz | Smoked Clams, Canned in Oil | 150 |
| 3 oz | Smoked Oysters, Canned in Oil | 150 |
| 1 cup | Smoked Whitefish | 150 |
| 3 oz | Sardines with Mustard, Canned | 165 |
| 3 oz | Shrimp, Breaded and Fried | 205 |
| 3 oz | Fish Cake, Breaded and Fried | 230 |
| 1 (3 oz) | Beef Patty, Broiled | 250 |

## Rice and Pasta

| Serving Size | Item | Calories |
|---|---|---|
| ½ cup | Wild Rice | 80 |
| ½ cup | Instant Brown Rice | 95 |
| ½ cup | Arrowhead Mills Brown Basmati Rice | 100 |
| ½ cup | Fantastic Foods Jasmine Rice | 115 |
| ½ cup | Uncle Ben's Whole Grain Brown Rice | 115 |
| ½ cup | Fantastic Foods Basmati White Rice | 120 |
| ½ cup | Rice-a-Roni Long Grain and Wild Rice | 120 |
| 1 cup | Bulgur | 150 |
| ½ cup | Rice-a-Roni Fried Rice | 160 |
| 1 cup | Couscous | 175 |
| 1 cup | Whole Wheat Pasta | 175 |
| 1 cup | Spinach Pasta | 185 |
| 1 cup | Tabbouleh | 185 |
| 1 cup | Pearled Barley | 195 |
| 1 cup | Macaroni | 200 |
| 1 cup | Egg Noodles | 215 |
| 1 cup | Millet | 280 |
| 1 cup | Lipton Pasta and Sauce (Cheddar Cheese and Broccoli) | 340 |

## Sauces, Condiments, and Marinades

| Serving Size | Item | Calories |
|---|---|---|
| 1 tsp | Capers | 0 |
| 1 Tbsp | Horseradish | 5 |

| | | |
|---|---|---:|
| 1 Tbsp | Worcestershire Sauce | 5 |
| 1 Tbsp | Barbecue Sauce | 10 |
| 1 Tbsp | Fat-Free Mayonnaise | 10 |
| 1 Tbsp | Healthy Choice Ketchup | 10 |
| 1 Tbsp | Kikkoman Lite Soy Sauce | 10 |
| 1 Tbsp | A-1 Steak Sauce | 15 |
| 1 Tbsp | Butter Buds | 15 |
| 1 Tbsp | Cocktail Sauce | 15 |
| 1 Tbsp | Dijon Mustard | 15 |
| 1 Tbsp | Ketchup | 15 |
| 1 Tbsp | Molly McButter | 15 |
| 1 Tbsp | Tamari Sauce | 15 |
| 1 Tbsp | Chili Sauce | 20 |
| 1 Tbsp | Pickle Relish | 20 |
| 1 Tbsp | Chutney | 25 |
| 1 Tbsp | Hellmann's Low-Fat Mayonnaise | 25 |
| 1 Tbsp | Sour Cream | 25 |
| 2 Tbsp | Kikkoman Stir-Fry Sauce | 30 |
| 2 Tbsp | LaChoy Duck Sauce | 45 |
| 5 | Kalamata Olives | 55 |
| ½ cup | Chi-Chi's Enchilada Sauce | 60 |
| ½ cup | Hunt's Ready Italian Sauce | 60 |
| ½ cup | Libby's Sloppy Joe Sauce | 70 |
| 1 Tbsp | Tartar Sauce | 70 |
| ½ cup | Curry Sauce | 75 |

*(continued)*

## Sauces, Condiments, and Marinades—continued

| Serving Size | Item | Calories |
|---|---|---|
| ½ cup | Barilla Mushroom and Garlic Pasta Sauce | 80 |
| ½ cup | Laury's Lemon Pepper Marinade | 80 |
| ½ cup | Progresso Red Clam Sauce | 80 |
| ½ cup | Progresso White Clam Sauce | 90 |
| 1 Tbsp | Mayonnaise | 100 |
| 2 Tbsp | Pesto Sauce | 155 |
| ½ cup | Contadina Light Alfredo Sauce | 160 |
| ½ cup | White Sauce | 200 |
| ½ cup | Cheese Sauce | 240 |
| ½ cup | Béarnaise Sauce | 320 |
| ½ cup | Alfredo Sauce, Ready to Serve | 340 |
| ½ cup | Hollandaise Sauce | 340 |

## Snacks

| Serving Size | Item | Calories |
|---|---|---|
| 5 | Health Valley Whole Wheat Crackers | 50 |
| 5 | Saltine Crackers | 60 |
| 3 | Rice Cakes | 105 |
| 20 | Baked Tostitos | 110 |
| 5 (1 oz) | Hard Pretzels | 115 |
| 8 (1 oz) | Pepperidge Farm Sesame Snack Sticks | 150 |
| 15 (10 oz) | Potato Chips | 150 |
| 6 | Tortilla Chips | 150 |
| ½ cup | Dried Apricots | 155 |

| 1 cup | Low-Fat Chocolate Milk | 160 |
| 47 | Pistachios | 160 |
| 24 | Almonds | 170 |
| ½ cup | Pepperidge Farm Cheddar Goldfish | 180 |
| 1 (2 oz) | Soft Pretzel | 190 |
| 10 | Dried Dates | 230 |
| 1 cup | Low-Fat Flavored Yogurt | 250 |
| 1 bag | Jolly Time Light Microwave Popcorn | 300 |
| 1 bag | Regular Microwave Popcorn | 480 |

## Soups

| Serving Size | Item | Calories |
|---|---|---|
| 1 cup | Healthy Valley Corn and Vegetable | 70 |
| 1 cup | Healthy Valley Lentil | 90 |
| 1 cup | Healthy Request Vegetable | 100 |
| 1 cup | Healthy Valley Pasta Italiano | 100 |
| 1 cup | Healthy Choice Minestrone | 110 |
| 1 cup | Healthy Valley Garden Split Pea | 110 |
| 1 cup | Progresso Barley | 110 |
| 1 cup | Imagine Organic Creamy Butternut Squash | 120 |
| 1 cup | Nile Spice Minestrone | 140 |
| 1 cup | Progresso Lentil | 140 |
| 1 cup | Healthy Choice Garden Tomato | 160 |
| 1 cup | Progresso Corn Chowder | 180 |
| 1 cup | Cream of Chicken | 190 |
| 1 cup | Wonton Soup | 190 |

*(continued)*

## Soups—continued

| Serving Size | Item | Calories |
|---|---|---|
| 1 cup | Cream of Mushroom | 200 |
| 1 cup | Olde Cape Cod's Corn Chowder | 220 |
| 1 cup | Campbell's Chunky New England Clam Chowder | 240 |
| 1 cup | Fantastic Chili Olé | 260 |
| 1 cup | Lobster Bisque | 300 |

## Spreads

| Serving Size | Item | Calories |
|---|---|---|
| 1 Tbsp | Smucker's Light Strawberry Preserves | 10 |
| 1 Tbsp | Smucker's Low-Sugar Jam | 25 |
| 1 Tbsp | Apple Butter | 35 |
| 1 Tbsp | Polaner All Fruit | 40 |
| 1 Tbsp | Smucker's Regular Jam | 50 |
| 1 Tbsp | Hellmann's Sandwich Spread | 55 |
| 1 Tbsp | Molasses | 55 |
| 2 Tbsp | Cream Cheese | 100 |
| 1 Tbsp | Margarine | 100 |
| 1 Tbsp | Butter | 110 |
| 2 Tbsp | Jif Reduced-Fat Peanut Butter | 190 |
| 2 Tbsp | Peanut Butter | 190 |

# INDEX

Underlined page references indicate boxed text.

# Picture-Perfect Shopper's I.Q. Answers

## The Vinaigrette Fallacy and the Salad Dressing Rule of Thumb

2 Tbsp regular vinaigrette dressing **150 calories**
2 Tbsp low-fat Parmesan Ranch salad dressing **45 calories**

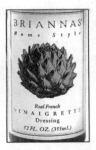

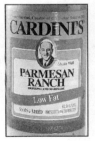

Call it the vinaigrette fallacy. Maybe it's the preeminence of the word *vinegar* in *vinaigrette*. Or perhaps it's that the vinaigrette looks clearer than the creamy ranch. Whatever the reason, we tend to think that the pure-looking, pungent vinaigrette dressing is calorie-free. In fact, however, a classic vinaigrette always contains three parts oil and one part vinegar; the oil alone gives this dressing a far greater calorie count than that of the low-fat, light dressing—despite the latter's creamy look and taste.

Where dressings are concerned, the savvy weight-conscious shopper should keep in mind this simple rule of thumb: Clear and liquidy dressings are not necessarily lower in calories.

## Comparison 2:
### Sugar Is Sugar Is Sugar

| | |
|---|---|
| 20-oz bottle regular cola | **250 calories** |
| 17.5-oz bottle unsweetened fruit juice | **264 calories** |
| 20-oz bottle naturally flavored sparkling water | **200 calories** |

From the point of view of Picture-Perfect Weight Loss, there's little to recommend any of these beverages, which are all high in calories. Don't be fooled by the claims of fruit or "natural" flavorings; the minuscule taste of fruit in these drinks is overpowered by their sugar content. (Not all flavored waters are high in calories; check the nutrition label.) The unsweetened fruit juice, at 17.5 ounces per bottle, actually contains more calories than the other two 20-ounce options! If it's fruit taste you want, eat a piece of fruit; the calories that you take in when you do will at least contain plenty of nutrients, with the added benefit of filling you up and satisfying your tastebuds. As an alternate, drink a low-calorie beverage.

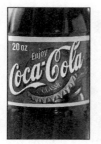 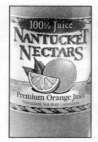 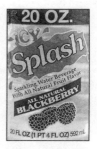

## Comparison 3:
### Challenging Assumptions

| | |
|---|---|
| 1 cup chicken /vegetable ramen noodle soup | **190 calories** |
| 1 cup black bean soup | **100 calories** |

Because the ramen soup comes in a small package and is of Japanese origin, we tend to assume it's a light, healthful soup with a low-calorie count. Because the bean soup is thick and hearty, we assume it's a high-calorie item. Both assumptions are wrong. The ramen soup, filled with saturated fat and starch, is twice as caloric as the bean soup. And the bean soup is far healthier—rich in protein, vitamins, minerals, and fiber.

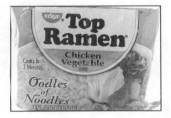

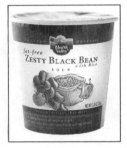

Visit Dr. Shapiro at www.drhowardshapiro.com